ACTIVE AND PASSIVE SMOKING HAZARDS IN THE WORKPLACE

ACTIVE AND PASSIVE SMOKING HAZARDS IN THE WORKPLACE

Judith A. Douville

VNR VAN NOSTRAND REINHOLD
New York

Library of Congress Catalog Card Number 89-24999
ISBN 0-442-00167-3

Printed in the United States of America

Van Nostrand Reinhold
115 Fifth Avenue
New York, New York 10003

Van Nostrand Reinhold International Company Limited
11 New Fetter Lane
London EC4P 4EE, England

Van Nostrand Reinhold
480 La Trobe Street
Melbourne, Victoria 3000, Australia

Nelson Canada
1120 Birchmount Road
Scarborough, Ontario M1K 5G4, Canada

16 15 14 13 12 11 10 9 8 7 6 5 4 3 2 1

Library of Congress Cataloging-in-Publication Data

Douville, Judith A.
Active and passive smoking hazards in the workplace
by Judith A. Douville.
p. cm.
Includes bibliographical references
ISBN 0-442-00167-3
1. Smoking—Health aspects. 2. Passive smoking—Health aspects.
3. Industrial hygiene. I. Title.
RA1242.T6D68 1990
616.86′5—dc20 89-24999
CIP

DEDICATION

To my father, Frank Peter Piliero, 1908–1986.

Preface

This non-medical book is designed to assist industrial, commercial, and government personnel directors, employee relations directors, safety and health managers, company or facility doctors, nurses and paraprofessionals, and public health officials in coping with the increased problems of workplace smoking. The book provides a practical guide, background information, and advice on the hazards of workplace smoking and passive exposure to environmental tobacco smoke. Ways of justifying enforcement of workplace smoking bans, both complete and partial, and discussions of and possible solutions to technical problems encountered while banning workplace smoking are presented.

The hazards of smoking, the nature of environmental tobacco smoke, and the effects of such smoke on the body are detailed. Special workplace hazards that become more dangerous when employees smoke, considerations for non-smoking co-workers and their need for clean air, health problems of smoking workers, air pollution from tobacco smoke, and the economic consequences of employees who smoke are treated. Smoking policies are reviewed and discussed, and smoking regulations for various workplace types are presented, along with state and federal workplace smoking regulations. This book is based largely on material provided by the U.S. Department of Health and Human Services.

Employer smoking intervention activities are presented, including programs for smoking cessation, smoking behavior modification, and other plans for modifying or stopping smoking in employees. Evaluations of several smoking cessation programs are also included.

Reader comments and suggestions will be appreciated and welcomed.

I thank, in this little paragraph, friends who helped make this volume possible. Harvey Satty provided able editorial leadership at Van Nostrand Reinhold, and Gene Falken asked me to take on this project. And, for making me aware of the problems of smoking, I thank friends, relatives, and a daughter, all of whom still smoke. Last, but not least, I am grateful for the patience, understanding, and unfailing support of my husband Phillip.

Contents

ACTIVE AND PASSIVE SMOKING HAZARDS IN THE WORKPLACE

1

Active and Passive Smoking: The Hazards

Involuntary, or "passive" smoking, as well as voluntary, or "active" smoking by persons in the workplace are a social and health problem. Persons not in their homes while smoking have social responsibilities toward other persons who may be inhaling the combusted tobacco products from cigarette, pipe, or cigar smoke. Many of these involuntary smokers have special health problems which may be made more acute by inhalation of combusted tobacco products, or environmental tobacco smoke (ETS). This book addresses the rights of persons to have clean air in the workplace, and to not be made ill by ETS from smokers, who also have rights. This book is designed to assist personnel in charge of workplace rights, and especially those rights in jeopardy because of smoking in the workplace.

The 1986 Report of the U.S. Surgeon General, *Health Consequences of Involuntary Smoking,* stated three major conclusions concerning smoking:

1. Involuntary smoking is a cause of disease, including lung cancer, in healthy nonsmokers.
2. Children of parents who smoke compared with children of nonsmoking parents have an increased frequency of respiratory infections, increased respiratory symptoms, and slightly smaller rates of increase in lung function as the lung matures.
3. Simple separation of smokers and nonsmokers within the same air space may reduce, but does not eliminate, the exposure of nonsmokers to environmental tobacco smoke.[1]

Hazards of smoking for active smokers, are numerous; researchers have listed chronic lung disease, including chronic bronchitis, and emphysema; cardiovascular diseases, including coronary heart disease, peripheral vascular disease, angina pectoris, and hypertension; and other disorders, including acute bronchitis, recurrent respiratory infections, asthma, hypercholesteremia, peptic ulcer, allergies, risk to pregnancy, and synergy with other agents. Smoking has been implicated in lung cancer, bladder cancer, cancer of the esophagus, and cancer of the larynx.

Passive, or involuntary smoking, also has associated health hazards; among these researchers have listed tissue irritation of eyes, throat, nose and airways; cardiovascular disease; pneumonia, chronic obstructive lung disease, chronic cough, and other respiratory symptoms, including tracheitis, laryngitis, and bronchitis; chronic ear effusions; and lung cancer. An obvious side effect of involuntary smoking is the worsening or aggravation of respiratory allergies, such as asthma or rhinitis. In a study conducted in Germany and reported in 1985, health risks posed by exposure to cigarette smoking in the workplace were studied. Evidence was presented to support the contention that cigarette smoking in the workplace caused more disease and death than all other occupational illnesses combined. Sidestream smoke, the portion inhaled by nonsmokers, was found to contain relatively higher levels of toxic substances than the smoke inhaled during active smoking. The carcinogenicity of passive smoke was proven conclusively in animal studies. Data from epidemiological studies revealed an increased risk of lung cancer among individuals passively exposed to cigarette smoke. In addition to the increased risk of cancer posed by exposure to cigarette smoke in the workplace, the acute effects of passive smoke, including burning eyes, cough, hoarseness, headaches, and genuine illness, in sensitive individuals were considered to be "bodily harm." The study concluded that smoking should be prohibited in the workplace and company doctors should help employees to stop smoking.[2]

HEALTH EFFECTS FROM TOBACCO SMOKE EXPOSURE

(There is ample evidence that nonsmokers are exposed to the elements of tobacco smoke when they are around people who are smoking. "Sidestream" smoke (which comes from the lit end of a cigarette, cigar, or pipe), smoke that escapes from the nonburning end) and mainstream smoke that has been inhaled by smokers and then exhaled, all mix with air in enclosed spaces to form "environmental tobacco smoke." "Passive smoking," "involuntary smoking," and "exposure to environmental tobacco smoke" are used synonymously in the literature to describe this phenomenon. Environmental tobacco smoke is basically the same, though lower in concentration, as the mixture to which smokers are exposed. Most lung cancer and chronic obstructive lung disease, as well as a large proportion of heart disease deaths, are clearly associated with active smoking, and tobacco smoke contains a number of substances that cause cancer in animals. These facts have led to continuing research to characterize the effects of environmental tobacco smoke on nonsmokers and on some particular groups that might be especially sensitive.

The most widespread acute effects of exposure to environmental tobacco smoke are eye irritation and irritation of the mucous membranes. Headaches and coughs are also commonly reported. These conditions are not life threatening or fatal, but large numbers of people, including smokers, experience them, some severely. There is little formal research on these acute effects, but they are often tangentially noted in reports of experimental research in this area, and are generally accepted as the result of environmental tobacco smoke exposure. It is therefore appropriate to consider them in developing smoking policies for the workplace.

The case is less clear regarding the contribution of passive smoking to chronic diseases. Debate about the link between passive smoking and lung cancer is one of the most contentious in public health today, and a similar contention has arisen about a possible link with heart disease. The other major category of concern is chronic obstructive lung disease. Because of documented exposure of nonsmokers to the constituents of tobacco smoke and the strong links of active smoking with these chronic diseases, the case for a connection with passive smoking achieves a measure of biological plausibility. Epidemiologic studies have been aimed at characterizing the extent to which these diseases are associated with passive smoking in the population. It has been estimated that, on the average, nonsmokers may inhale the tobacco smoke equivalent of one or two cigarettes per day. Three epidemiological studies have shown a significantly increased risk of lung cancer in nonsmokers passively exposed to cigarette smoke. In the workplace, passive exposure to cigarette smoke may result in significant smoke intake. It is noted that for nonsmokers in the same workplace with smokers, the workplace should be considered hazardous.[3]

There is currently a small amount of literature on the effects of passive smoking on the risk of developing chronic obstructive lung disease or heart disease. Some evidence suggests that long-term passive smoking by adults may result in decreased lung capacity. Experimental studies measuring short-term changes in lung function in response to environmental tobacco smoke lend support to this finding.[4] Evidence linking passive smoking to heart disease and cardiovascular symptoms is rather scanty, but studies suggest an acute exacerbation of anginal pain and an increased risk of death from cardiovascular disease. There has been found to be an increase in mortality from ischemic heart disease due to involuntary smoking.[5] Further research should clarify the role of passive smoking in causing and exacerbating these diseases.

More than a dozen studies have been published during the 1980s that address the possible association of passive smoking and lung cancer. Taken individually, the studies cannot be considered "definitive"; however, most investigators have found that passive smoking elevates a nonsmoker's risk of lung cancer, and results in about half the studies were statistically significant. The consistency of the results argues for stronger conclusions than could be drawn from individual studies: examined together, the evidence is generally consistent with an increased risk of lung cancer, on the order of a doubling of risk, among nonsmokers regularly exposed to environmental cigarette smoke compared to nonsmokers without exposure. These studies do not have the methodological strength of studies of direct smoking and lung cancer, and they cannot be interpreted without considering the effects on their results of potential biases. Despite the remaining uncertainties, the data are sufficient to warrant serious concern. Given the large number of people exposed, even a small increase in the risk of lung cancer from passive smoking would be important.

In summary, the evidence for an association of passive smoking with lung cancer has accumulated during the 1980s, and the evidence is consistent with the biologically plausible hypothesis that passive exposure to tobacco smoke can cause cancer. There is evidence that environmental tobacco smoke is an acute respiratory irritant in healthy adults. People with preexisting heart or lung disease can be especially sensitive to the effects of passive smoking.

NATURE OF ENVIRONMENTAL TOBACCO SMOKE: TOXICITY, ACUTE IRRITANT EFFECTS, AND CARCINOGENICITY

Irritants in Environmental Tobacco Smoke

Tobacco smoke is a complex aerosol that contains several thousand different constituents. Little is known about the health effects of most of these compounds individually, and even less is known about their collective action. Tobacco smoke contains compounds characterized as irritants, toxins, mutagens, and carcinogens. (The main irritants identified in ETS are respirable particulates, certain aldehydes, phenol, ammonia, nitrogen oxides, sulfur dioxide, and toluene.) The range of concentrations of these compounds measured in mainstream smoke, sidestream smoke, and smoky air under various conditions, or as results of field studies is anywhere from 1 part per billion to 40 milligrams, and is summarized in the accompanying table.

The levels of irritants in air contaminated with ETS vary considerably. Some of this variation is due to differences in the number of cigarettes smoked, the amount of ventilation, the adsorptive properties of the surroundings, and measurement methods. Researchers comparing the concentrations of these irritants with workplace air standards found that levels were in excess of those permitted for maximum emission concentrations for outdoor air pollutants such as respirable particulates, nitrogen dioxide, and acrolein. Other irritants generally do not reach existing threshold limit values under realistic conditions. An evaluation of the hygienic and medical importance of compounds in ETS is flawed because threshold values are established for healthy adults with an 8-hour exposure per day; other exposure values are for outdoor exposures only, and no indoor standards exist for ordinary conditions. Threshold limit

Table 1-1.
Major irritants in environmental tobacco smoke (ETS), their concentrations in mainstream smoke (MS), sidestream smoke (SS) to mainstream smoke (MS) ratios, and levels in smoky air under realistic and natural conditions[1]

Irritant	MS (per cigarette)	SS/MS (ratio)	Smoky air (range)
Acrolein	10–140μ	10–20	6–120 ppb
Formaldehyde	20–90μ	about 50	30–60 ppb[a] (CO: 1–43 ppb)
Ammonia	10–500μ	44–100	1000–4580 ppb[b]
Nitrogen oxides	16–600μ	4.7–50	1–370 ppb NO[c] 0–50 ppb NO_2[c]
Pyridine	32μ	10	NA[d]
Sulfur dioxide	1–75 ppb	NA	1–69 ppb[c]
Phenol	20–150μ	2.6	7.4–115 μ/m3
Toluene	108μ	5.6	0.04–1.04 mg/m3
Respirable particulates	0.1–40 mg	1.3–1.9	55–962 mg/m3

[a] Measured under experimental conditions only
[b] 1979 value
[c] Difference: indoor concentration minus control value (unoccupied room or outdoors)
[d] NA = not available

values are valid only for single compounds; (ETS contains many different irritants, which might interact to produce more toxicity than anticipated from the concentrations of individual compounds.)

Many of the constituents of tobacco smoke are also produced by other sources that contribute contaminants to indoor or outdoor environments; for instance, sources unrelated to smoking such as urea-formaldehyde foam insulation or certain wood products can emit formaldehyde and may give rise to mean air concentrations as high as 100 to 400 ppb. In measuring the contribution of tobacco smoke to the levels of these constituents, some researchers have subtracted the measured indoor concentrations from the levels measured either in unoccupied rooms or in outdoor environments near the rooms.

The measured concentrations of irritants listed in Table 1-1 are primarily the mean values in air samples collected over intervals of one-half hour to several hours. Substantial variation in levels can occur, depending on the proximity to a smoker and the air mixing conditions in a room. Peak concentrations of 3,300 to 99,680 nanograms/m^3 for particulates, and 41 to 750 ppb for nitrogen oxides in the "blowing cloud" 1 meter from the smoker immediately after smoke exhalation have been measured. These high concentrations decrease rapidly with time (half-life between 2 and 20 seconds) and distance from the smoker. Formaldehyde and acrolein concentrations have been measured at up to three orders of magnitude above occupational limits for more extended exposures to the sidestream smoke plume rising from a cigarette between puffs.

Irritating and Annoying Effects of Environmental Tobacco Smoke

The main effects of ETS irritants occur in the conjunctiva of the eyes and in the mucous membranes of the nose, throat, and lower respiratory tract. The main ocular symptoms are reddening, itching, and increased tearing; the main respiratory tract symptoms are itching, cough, and sore throat. The relationship of the site affected by ETS to the water solubility of the irritants has been demonstrated; the most water soluble irritants affect the eyes, larynx, and trachea; as water solubility decreases, irritants penetrate further into the respiratory tract, and bronchia, bronchioles, alveoli, and capillaries are ultimately affected by deep penetration of sulfur and nitrogen oxides, and respirable particulates. Particulates penetrate most deeply because their size in ETS is smaller than 1 micrometer, enabling them to penetrate the smallest airways.

Studies have shown that annoyance and irritation are the most common acute effects of ETS exposure. Of a group of persons reporting annoyance from ETS, 73% of nonsmokers were disturbed by restaurant smoking and 53% by office smoking. The most frequently reported symptom was eye irritation. Complaints of nausea, dizziness, and wheezing as well as runny nose were also reported, although much less often than stinging eyes. Similar results were obtained in a survey conducted in Europe; most complained about eye irritation. A survey of office workers found that nearly one-fourth of the nonsmokers reacted to smoke exposure with frustration and hostility.

A study conducted in 1980 of employees in 44 worksites (in 7 different firms, which included offices, design rooms, technical and clerical work areas, and conference rooms) measured carbon monoxide, nitrogen oxide, acrolein, particulates, and nicotine in room air before and during work times. Measurements were made in each room on 2 successive days and 472 employees were questioned about irritation and annoyance as well as about their opinions on involuntary smoking. Comparison of concentrations of pollutants due to smoking with concentrations due to measured absolute indoor concentrations revealed that 30 to 70% of measured indoor carbon monoxide, nitrogen oxide, and particulates were due to ETS. Approximately one-third of the workers described the air quality at work as "bad" with regard to tobacco smoke; 40% were disturbed by smoke; one-fourth reported eye irritation at work. Most significant was that 72% of the interviewed nonsmokers and 67% of the smokers were in favor of a separation of workrooms into smoking and nonsmoking sections, and 49% supported a partial or total prohibition of workplace smoking.

Not all studies have been as anti-smoking as the previous study; another researcher found no relationship between smoking conditions in offices and comfort complaints. Symptoms resembling those that were found to be related to ETS were similar in environments with and without smoking. However, no objective indoor air pollution measurements were made, and there were no descriptions of building ventilation. A "building illness" index was used that took account of several different symptoms in addition to irritation; and the irritating effects on the eye, the most sensitive organ, may have been masked by the use of this overall symptom index.

Acute physiological effects of ETS have been measured in healthy subjects; subjective eye irritation and mean eye blink rate increased with increasing smoke concentration. Annoyance increased rapidly as soon as smoke production began and increased with increasing smoke concentration. Evidently, objective irritant responses occur in healthy adults at smoke levels substantially lower than those in which airway responses are demonstrated. Research has indicated that the irritating effects of tobacco smoke are due to the semivolatile irritant compounds which volatize rapidly during tobacco combustion, recondense on particulates upon cooling, and deposit irritants in relatively high concentrations on mucous membranes.

EFFECTS OF ENVIRONMENTAL TOBACCO SMOKE

Effects on Special Individuals

Effect of ETS on children have indicated that 81% of 13-year old children disliked involuntary smoking and 82% complained of one or more kinds of irritation, mostly eye irritation. Several epidemiological studies have shown that children with parents who smoke have an increased risk for respiratory illness. Allergic individuals report tobacco smoke irritation more frequently than healthy individuals; persons at work and suffering from hay fever report significantly more eye irritation at work than those without this allergy.

Effects on the Lung

Cigarette smoking is associated with prominent changes in the numbers, types, and functions of respiratory epithelial and inflammatory cells. These alterations have been implicated in the development of pulmonary emphysema, chronic bronchitis, and respiratory tract cancers and in an increased susceptibility to infections. Chronic exposure to environmental tobacco smoke might cause similar changes. Because studies that directly address the effect of chronic exposure to ETS on lung structure have not been made, a review is given here of those studies in humans and animals that provide evidence on smoke exposures that may be relevant to ETS exposure.

Effects on the Respiratory Epithelium

Extensive evidence shows that exposure to cigarette smoke has adverse effects on respiratory epithelial cells, and dose-response relationships have been established for these changes. Studies involving the systematic examination of the bronchial mucosa from large numbers of human smokers have recorded three types of epithelial changes: epthelial hyperplasia, loss of cilia, and nuclear atypia. In autopsy studies of 402 adult males, 98% of the sections of tracheal and bronchial epithelium of the smokers had epithelial changes. The most common abnormality observed was atypical nuclei, and a large proportion of sections examined had hyperplasia. Denudation of the ciliated epithelium was also present in smokers. Similar relationships have been noted of smoking habits to laryngeal lesions, although the bronchial lesions appear to be more frequent and more advanced than those of the larynx.

The frequency and severity of epithelial lesions observed in smokers contrast sharply with those in persons who do not smoke regularly. In the autopsied smokers, 98% of the observed tracheobronchial sections had abnormalities; only 16.8% of nonsmokers had similar abnormal changes. The most common lesion noted in nonsmokers was epithelial hyperplasia; atypical cells were seen in only 4.8% of sections from nonsmokers. Therefore, it seems reasonable to assume that persons chronically exposed to ETS will have changes in respiratory epithelial cells.[6]

Cigarette smoking also has adverse effects on the bronchial wall beneath the epithelium. Submucosal gland atrophy has been observed frequently; the prevalence is related to the intensity of cigarette smoking. This disorder is noted in nonsmokers, but not very often. The loss of ciliary epithelium, increased numbers of goblet cells, and mucous gland hypertrophy frequently observed in smokers would predict mucociliary dysfunction. Available evidence suggests that long-term cigarette smoking impairs mucociliary transport. Once a cigarette smoker develops chronic bronchitis, mucus transport appears to be irreversibly damaged, and impairment persists even in persons who have abstained from smoking for many years.

Effects on Lung Inflammatory Cells

One of the earliest pathologic lesions found in the lungs of young smokers is a respiratory bronchiolitis. Clusters of pigment-laden phagocytes lodge in the respiratory bronchioles of smokers precisely at the sites of the earliest lung injury. The infiltration of these phagocytes, predominantly alveolar macrophages, precedes the development of emphysema and focal fibrosis. Lung fluid yields of alveolar macrophages are 5 to 7 times greater for smokers than for nonsmokers. The alveolar macrophages from smokers appear to be activated both morphologically and metabolically; their altered function and location have led to the hypothesis that they may contribute to the alteration of enzyme balances in the lower respiratory tract, ultimately leading to emphysema.

The influence of cigarette smoking on many aspects of the human immune system has been studied; immunoglobin levels in the peripheral blood of smokers has been reported to be decreased according to some studies. Cell-mediated immunity may also be affected by smoking, and natural killer-cell activity in the blood of smokers appears to be decreased. Smoking modifies the immune response to inhaled antigens.[7]

The extent to which alterations of lung inflammatory cell numbers and functions observed in smokers are also present in persons chronically exposed to ETS remains unknown. However, the characteristic inflammatory lesions seen in the lungs of smokers are usually absent or modest in persons who do not smoke cigarettes and who are not exposed to alternative causative agents.

Effects on Lung Parenchyma

The most striking alteration of lung parenchyma associated with cigarette smoking is centrilobular emphysema. The relationship between smoking history, age, and degree of emphysema have been studied; the effect of smoking on the development of emphysema is believed to be cumulative. The extent of emphysema strongly correlates with the number of cigarettes smoked daily; emphysema is rare in individuals who do not smoke regularly and do not have a genetic predisposition for the disease. Histological examination showed that the lungs of all smokers contained enlarged air spaces and varying degrees of interstitial fibrosis. Emphysema scores in smokers were higher than in nonsmokers and increased with heavy cigarette smoking. In contrast, lungs of nonsmokers showed a uniform age-related enlargement of air spaces with no significant fibrosis. There is a smoking associated increase in the elemental dust load of aluminum and silicon in the lungs of cigarette smokers. There is also a clear relationship between smoking and the development of emphysema.[8]

The prevalence of radiologically detectable parenchymal small opacities in workers with shorter exposure times was higher in smokers. No such association was observed for pleural changes. Possible mechanisms for smoking effects might be interference with alveolar clearing mechanisms, effect on macrophages, or other cellular and humoral factors.[9]

Carcinogenicity of Environmental Tobacco Smoke

Chemical analytical studies have demonstrated that sidestream smoke and ETS contain a wide spectrum of carcinogens including polynuclear aromatic hydrocarbons, volatile and tobacco-specific N-nitrosamines, and polonium-210. Animal studies have demonstrated the carcinogenicity of ETS, and the limited data that exist suggest that more carcinogenic activity per milligram of cigarette smoke concentrate may be contained in sidestream smoke than in mainstream (inhaled) cigarette smoke. A study done as far back as 1961 noted that cigarette smoking was a major factor in the causation of bronchogenic carcinoma.[10]

REFERENCES

1. *Health Consequences of Involuntary Smoking: A Report of the Surgeon General.* U.S. Department of Health and Human Services, Public Health Service. Washington, DC: Superintendent of Documents, U.S. Government Printing Office, 1986. 359 pp. DHHS(CDC)87-8398. pp. 7, 21–28, 132–147, 164–169, 181–198, 229–252, 265–308.

2. Schmidt, F. "Smoking in the workplace,"*Zentralblatt fur Arbeitsmedizin* 35(11), 352–355, 1985. (NIOSH-00167409)

3. Benowitz, N.L. "Smoking and occupational lung cancer," *Cancer Prevention: Strategies in the Workplace,* edited by C.E. Becker and M.J. Coye. Washington, DC: Hemisphere Publ., 1986, pp. 121–142. (NIOSH-00170820)

4. Dahms, T.E., J.F. Bolin, and R.G. Slavin. "Passive smoking," *Chest* 80(5), 530–534, 1981. (NIOSH-00126844)

5. Garland, C., E. Barrett-Connor, L. Suarez, M.H. Criqui, and D.L. Wingard. "Effects of passive smoking on ischemic heart disease mortality of nonsmokers: A prospective study," *American Journal of Epidemiology* 121(5), 645–650, 1985. (NIOSH-00147182)

6. Huchon, G.J., J.A. Russell, L.G. Barritault, A. Lipavsky, and J.F. Murray. "Chronic air-flow limitation does not increase respiratory epithelial permeability assessed by aerosolized solute, but smoking does," *American Review of Respiratory Disease* 130(3), 457–460, 1984. (NIOSH-00144427)

7. Terho, E.O., K. Husman, I. Vohlonen, and R.A. Mantyjarvi. "Serum precipitins against microbes in mouldy hay with respect to age, sex, atopy, and smoking of farmers," *Journal of Respiratory Diseases* 71, Supplement No. 152 (Work-Related Respiratory Diseases Among Finnish Farmers), 115–121, 1987. (NIOSH-00174605)

8. Vallyathan, V., and L.H. Hahn. "Cigarette smoking and inorganic dust in human lungs," *Archives of Environmental Health* 40(2), 69–73, 1985. (NIOSH-00151224)

9. Lilis, R., I.J. Selikoff, Y. Lerman, H. Siedman, and S.K. Gelb. "Asbestosis: Interstital pulmonary fibrosis and pleural fibrosis in a cohort of asbestos insulation workers: Influence of cigarette smoking," *American Journal of Industrial Medicine* 10(5/6), 459–470, 1986. (NIOSH-00164996)

10. Auerbach, O., A.P. Stout, E.C. Hammond, and L. Garfinkel. "Changes in bronchial epithelium in relation to cigarette smoking and in relation to lung cancer," *New England Journal of Medicine* 265, 253–267, Aug. 10, 1961. (NIOSH-0086218)

2

Workplace Hazards of Smoking

Smoking in the workplace, either voluntarily or involuntarily, may have special hazards caused by the nature of the workplace. Workers involved with chemicals may be placed at risk because of the health hazards of the chemicals themselves, plus the added synergistic risk of ETS. This chapter discusses, in addition to the health hazards of tobacco smoke, various workplace hazards, work risk situations, and other considerations which when coupled with smoking may place workers at serious health risk.

CONCERNS OF COMMERCIAL EMPLOYERS

Employers, for the most part, will try to make the workplace comfortable and safe for employees, so that work can be done with a minimum of distraction. Such considerations as ventilation and heating (if these functions use the same ductwork and air supply), for instance, will affect the speed and range of air pollution problems, such as that of ETS. ETS can and will be distributed by air venting equipment, so that a separate smoking area's ETS-laden air will be found throughout a building in a short time. The air systems in use must be rethought and redesigned if smoking is permitted within the workplace. The best arrangement when having a separate smoking area for employees is to ventilate and heat it separately so that the air supply of the smoking area does not intermix with those of the rest of the facility. The other solution to the ventilation/heating system problem is to prohibit smoking inside the building at all times. Some firms have forced smokers to smoke outdoors, regardless of the weather. Because the legislation now in force requiring workplace smoking regulations is so new, it is too early to tell if labor unions will require employers to install separate areas to spare workers their outdoor smoking breaks.

Other concerns of employers in non-office, or research and laboratory settings, are that employees are not unduly exposed to chemicals, with which ETS may have a synergistic effect. ETS-laden workplace air, combined with vapors in poorly ventilated chemical laboratories, presents at least a two-fold risk to employees, some of whom may also have allergies or respiratory problems. Laboratory ventilation may be adequate for chemical vapors, but the make-up air to the laboratory must also be smoke-free. Employees must never smoke in chemical laboratories, for a multitude of reasons; they should not have to breathe smoker's air, either.

Workers' physical condition and the amount of exercise obtained during the course of the workday will also be a factor when ETS-contaminated air is breathed. Involuntary smoking will, as will voluntary smoking, limit the breathing capacity of workers to some extent. A worker who has respiratory limitations of any type will not appreciate contaminated air over the course of the workday; indeed, polluted air will certainly exacerbate the worker's discomfort. ETS-contaminated air is irritating to normal respiratory area mucosa, and if workers cannot seek other air supplies (by changing work areas, for instance), they may become ill. Poor quality air can be psychologically irritating, as well; it is an annoyance that has no place in the normal workplace.

The ability to withstand contaminated air, especially ETS-contamination, varies with age, sex, physical fitness level, pregnancy/nonpregnancy, and with the presence of respiratory or cardiovascular disease. Workers being hired must obtain physical examinations from their physicians to ascertain their ability to perform certain jobs demanded during the course of their employment; however, in most instances, these examinations do not consider the ability to function while breathing smoke-filled air. Breathing tests that are given, for the most part, do not measure the body's reaction to air pollutants, and presume clean air to be the norm.

CONCERNS OF INDUSTRIAL EMPLOYERS

The industrial employer, in making the workplace comfortable for the employee, has special concerns which complicate the smoking-nonsmoking question. Workers in special industrial jobs, such as mining, toxic materials handling, firefighting, chemical industries, and the like, need special attention to their air supplies while at work. In some instances, such as that of the firefighter, the ambient air cannot be controlled, but the worker's personal smoking habits will need monitoring, lest they interfere with breathing functions and make the worker's job dangerous.

Various types of work situation present special problems when the question of smoking on the job is considered. The list of hazardous materials, made more hazardous due to synergy with ingested smoke and materials, is long; a list of problem job areas follows:

Asbestos	Sulfur dioxide
Silica	Polyvinyl chloride
Coal	Vinyl chloride
Petrochemicals	Smelting
Aromatic amines	Coating processes
Pesticides	Textiles
Cotton dust	Styrene
Ionizing radiation	Farm areas
Cement	Molds
Grain	Grains
Welding	Pesticide applications

CONCERNS OF SPECIAL EMPLOYERS

Certain employers do not fit into any of the categories cited above, but have special concerns about air quality in their workplaces. Among these are laboratories where biological research is performed, or where chemical experimentation takes place; clean rooms, where operations are performed using extremely pure substances that must be contamination-free; and hospitals, that have patients who may not have resistance to poor air, and where staff must spend long hours ministering to possibly unhealthy persons. In this last category fall hospital operating rooms, which generate their own type of pollution: waste anesthetic gases.

WHAT CONSTITUTES PASSIVE EXPOSURE TO TOBACCO SMOKE?

It has been rather easy to approximate relative exposure levels among smokers to cigarette smoke as the number of cigarettes smoked per day and the number of years that the person has smoked. Quantifying passive exposure of nonsmokers to cigarette smoke is more difficult. One part of the effort to characterize exposure of nonsmokers has been to measure the concentrations of cigarette smoke constituents in indoor environments and to determine the contributions of "sidestream" and "mainstream" smoke to "environmental" tobacco smoke. There have been about two dozen investigations of environmental tobacco smoke constituents, including both controlled studies in special experimental chambers and measurements in the air of smoky restaurants, bars, and nightclubs, and other smoky, enclosed spaces. A second and more recent thrust has been to test the body fluids—blood, urine, and saliva—of passively exposed nonsmokers for elevated levels of tobacco smoke constituents or their metabolites (smoke constituents modified within the body to become different chemical entities).

Mainstream, Sidestream, and Environmental Smoke

Mainstream smoke is the tobacco smoke that is generated during a puff and is drawn through the butt end into the smoker's respiratory system. Sidestream smoke comes directly from the burning end of the cigarette, cigar, or pipe. Environmental tobacco smoke refers to what passive smokers are actually exposed to. Smokers, of course, are exposed to both mainstream and environmental smoke.

A smoker's exposure results primarily from the mainstream smoke drawn into the lungs. Nonsmokers are exposed primarily to sidestream smoke (nearly 85% of the smoke in a room is sidestream smoke) and to smaller amounts of exhaled mainstream smoke, smoke that comes from the nonburning end of the cigarette but is not inhaled by the smoker, and smoke that diffuses through the paper wrapper of the cigarette.

Researchers have designed laboratory apparatus to measure the amounts of the various substances contained in sidestream and mainstream smoke. The instruments measure the concentrations in the smoke immediately after it leaves the butt end (mainstream smoke) or the burning end (sidestream smoke) of the cigarette. Measured in this fashion, the concentrations of many toxic substances in captured sidestream smoke are greater than those found in mainstream smoke, e.g., tar, nicotine, benzo[a]pyrene.[1] This is because different amounts of tobacco are burned when producing mainstream and sidestream smoke, the tobacco's burning temperature is different during puffing compared to when it is only smoldering, and some substances are absorbed by the tobacco and filter as the mainstream smoke passes through.

Because smoke is diluted by air in a room, the exposures of nonsmokers are much less than the measured concentrations of toxic substances in sidestream or mainstream smoke as they emerge directly from the cigarette. In addition to the effects of dilution, environmental tobacco smoke differs somewhat from mainstream and sidestream smoke as a result of chemical and physical changes that occur as mainstream and sidestream smoke cool and react in the air. A number of researchers over the years have documented the significant contribution of environmental tobacco smoke to indoor air pollution in studies of enclosed spaces. For example, the largest particles in sidestream smoke tend to settle out of the air and some gases react to form different substances. While the differences between what smokers and nonsmokers are exposed to have been frequently emphasized, they are not so great as to require a conclusion that sidestream smoke is dramatically different from mainstream smoke.

Measurements of Specific Constituents of Environmental Tobacco Smoke

More than 2000 constituents of environmental tobacco smoke have been identified; many of these substances cause cancer in experimental animals. The National Research Council Committee on Indoor Pollution concluded that passive smoking constituted the "principal source of exposure to many of these compounds" for many people. The most frequently measured products of cigarette smoke in indoor air are carbon monoxide and particulates; other constituents such as dimethynitrosamine, benzo[a]pyrene, and nicotine, have been measured less frequently. Polonium-210, a radioactive isotope, is also present in environmental tobacco smoke. This literature is reviewed in the 1981 National Research Council study, *Indoor Pollutants,* and in the 1984 Surgeon General's *Report on Chronic Obstructive Lung Disease*.

Measurements of environmental tobacco smoke usually distinguish between the gaseous phase and the particulate phase; the latter consists not only of particles, but some other compounds that adhere to the particles. Investigations to characterize levels of exposure, rather than the makeup of the smoke, have chosen to measure one or more compounds thought to be representative of smoke levels. The appropriate constituents to measure differ for particulates, which tend to settle out of the air more quickly, and the gaseous phase, which remains in the air for relatively long periods. The characteristics of enclosed spaces, such as their size and particularly their ventilation, affect the fate of cigarette smoke and therefore the opportunity for passive exposure to smoke.

Carbon monoxide is an easily measured combustion product of burning tobacco, and the most frequently quantified component of the gaseous phase. Carbon monoxide is generated by sources of combustion other than burning tobacco, such as automobiles and gas cooking. The OSHA has set a workplace permissible exposure limit of 50 ppm, averaged over 8 hours. In 1972, NIOSH recommended a 10-hour average limit of 35 ppm, and their 8-hour standard, an average limit, is 9 ppm; both limits may be exceeded only once per year.

Carbon monoxide levels in areas where people have been smoking are consistently higher than in "control" areas, which can be outdoors in some cases or indoor spaces where there has been no smoking. Levels of between 10 ppm and 20 ppm often occur in areas such as nightclubs, taverns, and automobiles. Most measurements reported in restaurants are in the range of 5–10 ppm. Control levels range from 1–3 ppm.

Acrolein is the gaseous constituent responsible for most of the odor associated with cigarette smoke, and also may cause eye and throat irritation. Levels of acrolein found in enclosed spaces under conditions of heavy smoking have exceeded the levels recommended in industrial conditions.

Nicotine is found in both the gaseous phase and the particulate phase, and is technically difficult to measure. A few studies have quantified nicotine concentrations, however, showing significant increases over background levels.

A more common measurement has been of total particulates, which also are elevated in areas where people have been smoking.[2] In one study of 69 homes in 6 cities, average particulate concentrations were 43 micrograms per cubic meter of air in homes with one cigarette smoker; 75 micrograms per cubic meter in homes with two or more smokers; compared with 24 micrograms per cubic meter in homes with no smokers and 22 micrograms per cubic meter outdoors. Measures of total particulates may include a great deal of material not associated with tobacco smoke, however, and are influenced by a wide variety of factors, including the number of people in a room. A measure of total particulates, therefore, may not be as useful as some of the more specific indicators of the level of environmental tobacco smoke.

Other gaseous constituents that have been measured and found elevated in smoky conditions are nitrogen oxides, nitrosamines, carbon dioxide, methane, acetylene, ammonia, hydrogen cyanide, methylfuran, acetonitrile, and pyridine. Tar, water, toluene, phenol, methylnaphthalene, pyrene, benzo[a]pyrene, aniline, and naphthylamine, constituents of the particulate phase, are also elevated in smoky conditions.

Biologic Evidence of Passive Exposure to Tobacco Smoke

Certain constituents of tobacco smoke are measurable, some easily so, in the blood, urine, and saliva of smokers. These indicators have been used, for instance, to verify self-reported smoking status, especially among people who claimed to have stopped smoking. In nonsmokers, these same indicators have been used in a number of studies to estimate exposure levels of nonsmokers to varying amounts of ETS.

When carbon monoxide is inhaled, it enters the bloodstream via the lungs. Carbon monoxide has an extremely strong affinity for the hemoglobin molecules contained in red blood cells, more than 200 times stronger than the affinity of oxygen molecules for hemoglobin, and competes successfully with oxygen for carriage on the hemoglobin molecule. (At very high doses, carbon monoxide is lethal, as it displaces so much oxygen that the tissues become oxygen–starved.) The combination of carbon monoxide and hemoglobin is a molecule called "carboxyhemoglobin," which can be measured in blood. Studies have shown increases in carboxyhemoglobin after exposure to environmental tobacco smoke, which are, as expected, smaller than changes recorded after direct smoking. With a half life of about 4 hours in blood, carboxyhemoglobin is a good indicator of acute exposure to cigarette smoke (or other types of combustion), but is not a good indicator of chronic exposure.

Serum thiocyanate (SCN), the metabolite of hydrogen cyanide, a constituent of tobacco smoke, has also been used to verify self-reported smoking status, and has been used in a few studies of nonsmokers' environmental smoke exposure. The value of SCN measurements is limited by many factors, unrelated to smoke exposure, that influence levels of thiocyanate in the blood.

Nicotine is the most tobacco-specific constituent in smoke that occurs in relatively large quantities. It is possible to measure nicotine in body fluids, but its half-life of about 30 minutes makes nicotine unsuitable for estimating chronic exposure. Nicotine has been measured in the blood, urine, and saliva of nonsmokers under both experimental and in typical workplace conditions. Under workplace conditions, researchers found that all nonsmokers had detectable levels of nicotine in saliva and urine. Those nonsmokers who reported exposure to cigarette smoke had significantly higher levels than those who reported no exposure. There was some overlap of nicotine levels of exposed nonsmokers and levels in light smokers in the sample (smokers who have smoked three or fewer cigarettes before the sample was taken), but most of the overlap was with smokers who had not yet smoked a cigarette on the day the urine sample was taken.

Cotinine appears to be the most promising marker of passive smoke exposure. Cotinine, the major metabolite of nicotine, has a half life of 20–30 hours, so consistent, daily exposure to tobacco smoke should result in elevated levels of cotinine as measured in blood, urine, or saliva. Cotinine levels have been measured in the blood and urine of smokers since the late 1970s, and correlate well with levels of smoking. A recent study in smokers indicates good correlation of cotinine levels and nicotine content of cigarettes smoked, and of changes in smoking habits. That study also points out that cotinine levels in the urine, blood, and saliva may change at different rates over time and are not equally sensitive to changes in exposure.

Recently, studies of urine cotinine in nonsmokers have been carried out in attempts to measure passive exposure to cigarette smoke. Researchers found higher levels of urinary cotinine in Japanese nonsmokers passively exposed to tobacco smoke at home, at work, or in both locations, and the effects were dose related in both settings. They also compared cotinine levels in nonsmokers from rural areas with those in urban areas, and found that, for nonsmokers who did not live with smokers, levels were significantly lower for rural compared with urban dwellers. Nonsmokers with the highest urine cotinine levels were those exposed to the smoke of more than 40 cigarettes per day at home; those individuals had cotinine levels similar to those of smokers of up to three cigarettes per day.[3]

Summary: Characterizing Passive Exposure

There is no doubt that tobacco smoking indoors contributes chemical and physical components to the air that are qualitatively similar to the smoke taken into smokers' lungs. The levels of these constituents to which nonsmokers are exposed are much lower levels than those to which smokers are exposed, and the levels vary depending on the amount of smoking around the nonsmoker, the architecture and ventilation of the structure, other aspects of air quality (such as humidity), and chemical and physical changes that take place in the air. Nevertheless, the major components of tobacco smoke have been repeatedly detected in enclosed spaces in which there has been smoking, at higher levels than occur in the absence of smoking. Biologic measurements of tobacco smoke constituents and their metabolites in nonsmokers provide direct, convincing evidence that nonsmokers do have measurable internal exposure to environmental tobacco smoke, and that levels of exposure are related to the number of cigarettes and/or smokers to which they are exposed.

EXPOSURE TO ENVIRONMENTAL TOBACCO SMOKE: CONSTITUENTS

Radioactivity of Tobacco Smoke

Naturally occurring decay products of radon are found in tobacco and, therefore, also in tobacco smoke. These include the isotopes of lead (Pb-210), bismuth (Bi-210), polonium (Po-210), and radon, which originates from the decay of uranium through radium. Radon and its short-lived daughters (Po-218, Pb-214, Bi-214, Po-214), which precede long-lived daughters in the decay chain, are ubiquitous in indoor air and are largely derived from sources other than tobacco smoke. Most of the radon daughters are attached to particles in the air, but a small proportion are not.

It has been suggested that the presence of Pb-210 and subsequent decay products in tobacco is dependent upon an absorption of short-lived radon daughters on the leaves of the tobacco plant, especially where phosphate fertilizers which are rich in radium have been used and have caused increased leakage of radon from the ground. These attached short-lived radon daughters then decay to long-lived Pb-210 and subsequent nuclides found in the tobacco. However, the origin of these decay products may also depend on the general occurrence of radon in the atmosphere and not on the local emanation of radon.

In recent years, it has been shown that relatively high levels of radon and short-lived radon daughters may occur in indoor air, and consistent observations in this regard have been made in several countries. In the air with a very low concentration of particles, the proportion of unattached radon daughters is increased beyond that found with a higher concentration of particles. The unattached daughters are removed more rapidly than those which are attached by plating out on walls and fixtures. The addition of an aerosol, such as tobacco smoke, increases the attached fraction, elevates the concentration of radon daughters, and reduces the rate of removal of radon daughters. The dose of alpha radiation received by the airway epithelium depends not only on the concentration of radon daughters but also on the unattached fraction and on the size distribution of the inhaled particles. The interplay among these factors as they are modified by ETS has not yet been fully examined.

Environmental Tobacco Smoke

The air dilution of sidestream smoke, and of other contributors to ETS, causes several physicochemical changes in the aerosol. The concentration of particles in ETS depends on the degree of air dilution and may range from 300 to 500 mg/m^3 to a few micrograms/m^3. At the same time, the median diameter of particles may decrease as undiluted sidestream smoke is diluted to form ETS. Furthermore, nicotine volatilizes during air dilution of sidestream smoke, so that in ETS it occurs almost exclusively in the vapor phase. This is reflected in the fairly rapid occurrence of relatively high concentrations of nicotine in the saliva of people entering a smoke-polluted room. Most likely there are also redistributions between the vapor phase and the particulate phase of other constituents of sidestream smoke due to air dilution, which may account for the presence of other semivolatiles in the vapor phase of ETS.

Comparison of Toxic and Carcinogenic Agents in Mainstream Smoke and in Environmental Tobacco Smoke

The combustion products of cigarettes are the source of both ETS and mainstream smoke. Therefore, comparisons of the levels of specific toxins and carcinogens in ETS with the corresponding levels in the mainstream smoke are relevant to an estimation of the risk of ETS exposure. Although ETS is a far less concentrated aerosol than undiluted mainstream smoke, both inhalants contain the same volatile and nonvolatile toxic agents and carcinogens. This fact and the current knowledge about the quantitative relationships between dose and effect that are commonly observed from exposure to carcinogens have led to the conclusion that inhalation of ETS gives rise to some risk of cancer.

However, comparisons of ETS and mainstream smoke should include the consideration of differences between the two aerosols with regard to their chemical composition, including pH levels, and their physicochemical nature (particle size, air dilution factors, and distribution of agents between vapor phase and particulate phase). Another important consideration pertains to the differences between inhaling ambient air and inhaling a concentrated smoke aerosol during puff-drawing. Finally, chemical and physicochemical data established by the analysis of smoke generated by machine-smoking are certainly not fully comparable to the levels and characteristics of compounds generated when a smoker inhales cigarette smoke. This caveat applies particularly to the smoking of low-yield cigarettes, for which the yields of smoke constituents in machine-generated smoking and human smoking may be very different.

The assignment of various smoke constituents as human carcinogens, suspected human carcinogens, or animal carcinogens is based on definitions by the International Agency for Research on Cancer. Accordingly, a human carcinogen is an agent for which sufficient evidence of carcinogenicity indicates that there is a causal relationship between exposure and human cancer; a suspected human carcinogen is an agent for which limited evidence of carcinogenicity indicates that a causal interpretation is credible, but that alternate explanations could not adequately be excluded. An animal carcinogen is an agent for which there is sufficient evidence of carcinogenicity in animals, but for which no data on humans are available. Table 2-1 shows the toxic and carcinogenic constituents of ETS found in indoor environments.

Polonium-210 is not listed in this table because there are no

Table 2-1.
Concentrations of Toxic and Carcinogenic Agents in Nonfilter Cigarette Mainstream Smoke and in Environmental Tobacco Smoke (ETS) in Indoor Environments[d]

Agent	Weight	Mainstream Smoke Concentration
Carbon monoxide	10–23 mg	24,900–57,300 ppm
Nitrogen oxide	100–600 μg	230,000–1,400,000 ppb
Nitrogen dioxide	<5 μg	<7,600 ppb
Acrolein	60–100 μg	75,000–125,000 ppb
Acetone	100–250 μg	120,000–300,000 ppb
Benzene[b]	12–48 μg	11,000–43,000 ppb
N-Nitrosodimethylamine[c]	10–40 ng	9–38 ppb
N-Nitrosodiethylamine[c]	4–25 ng	3–17 ppb
Nicotine	1,000–2,500 ng	430,000–1,080,000 ppb
Benzo[a]pyrene (4)	20–40 ng	5–11 ppb

Note: Values for inhaled mainstream smoke components were calculated from values in Table 2 in Reference 4 and on a respiratory rate of 10 L per minute. Values for carbon monoxide and nicotine represent the range in mainstream smoke of U.S. nonfilter cigarettes as reported by the U.S. Federal Trade Commission (1985). Data under ETS are derived from tables 8-15 in that latter reference, with data from the unventilated interior compartments of automobiles excluded.

[a] The designation "episodic high values" was chosen to classify those data in the literature that require confirmation.

[b] Human carcinogen according to IARC and suspected carcinogen according to ACGIH (1985).

[c] Animal carcinogen according to IARC.

[d] Suspected human carcinogen according to IARC and ACGIH (1985).

data on the concentration of this isotope in ETS, although it is a component of both mainstream and sidestream smoke. Whereas in clean air the short-lived radon daughters tend to plate out on room surfaces, in the presence of some aerosol such as ETS, some of the short-lived radon daughters become attached to particles and consequently remain available for inhalation. Radon daughter background concentration may more than double in the presence of ETS. Other possible

Inhaled as ETS Constituents During 1 Hour			
Range		Episodic High Values	
Weight	Concentration	Weight	Concentration
1.2–22 mg	1–18.5 ppm	37 mg	32 ppm
7–90 μ	9–120 ppb	146 μg	195 ppb
24–87 μ	21–76 ppb	120 μg	105 ppb
8–72 μ	6–50 ppb	110 μg	80 ppb
210–720 μ	150–500 ppb	3,500 μg	2,400 ppb
19–190 μ	6–98 ppb	190 μg	98 ppb
6–140 ng	0.003–0.072 ppb	140 ng	0.072 ppb
<6–120 μ	<0.002–0.05 ppb	120 ng	0.05 ppb
0.6–30 μ	0.15–7.5 ppb	300 μg	75 ppb
1.7–460 ng	0.0002–0.04 ppb	460 ng	0.04 ppb

carcinogens derived from ETS are cadmium, arsenic, lead, and zinc. Cigarettes are a major source of cadmium in humans and can contribute more to the total body burden than the amount derived from other sources.[5] Studies have revealed that smokers have higher concentrations of cadmium and lead in their blood than do subjects who do not smoke.[6,7,8,9]

Number and Size Distribution of Particles in Environmental Tobacco Smoke

ETS consists of the combined products of both fresh and aged sidestream smoke and exhaled mainstream smoke. Coagulation, evaporation, and particle removal on surfaces occur simultaneously to modify the physical characteristics of the ETS particles; as a result, the "typical" particle size and chemical composition of ETS may vary with age of the smoke and characteristics of the environment. Other factors such as relative humidity, particle concentration, and temperature may also affect ETS characteristics.

The rapid dilution of sidestream smoke as it is emitted into a room leads to a number of physical and chemical changes. For example, evaporation of volatile species as ETS ages reduces the median diameter of smoke particles. Studies have indicated that the mass median diameter of ETS is between 0.2 and 0.4 micrometer. ETS particles are in the diffusion-controlled regime for particle removal and therefore will tend to follow stream lines, remain airborne for long periods of time, and rapidly disperse through open volumes.

A number of factors can produce variations in the mean size of the particles in ETS; however, in considering transport, deposition, and removal in the human lung, it is useful to assume that the particle sizes of aged ETS will generally be between 0.1 and 0.4 micrometer. Although it is not possible to assign a single value for the diameter of sidestream smoke particles, the difference in deposition efficiency in the human respiratory tract between 0.2 and 0.4 micrometer particles is negligible. Particles in this size range are not efficiently removed by sedimentation or impaction. Although diffusion is the major removal mechanism for particles of this size, it is minimally efficient in the 0.2–0.4 micrometer range. The relatively low particle deposition efficiency for sidestream smoke particles in human volunteers observed in a controlled study is consistent with particles in this size range.

Studies have shown that techniques using similar instruments provide similar results for size distribution of both sidestream and mainstream particles. However, the chemical composition of the mainstream and sidestream smoke particles can be quite different because of the very different conditions of their generation, and the subsequent dilution and aging that ETS undergoes before inhalation.

Estimating Human Exposure to Environmental Tobacco Smoke

Human exposure to ETS can be estimated by using approaches similar to those used for other airborne pollutants. The concentration of ETS to which an individual is exposed depends on factors such as the type and number of cigarettes smoked, the volume of the room, the ventilation rate, and the proximity to the source. These factors, along with the duration of exposure and individual characteristics such as ventilatory rate and breathing pattern, influence the dosage received by an individual.

Ideally, the health effects of exposures to ETS might be assessed by quantifying the time dependent exposure dose for each of the several thousand compounds in cigarette smoke and defining the dose response relationships for these compounds in producing disease, both as isolated compounds and in various combinations. The magnitude of this task, given the number of compounds in smoke, and the limited knowledge of the precise mechanisms by which these compounds cause disease, have led to a simpler approach, one that attempts to use measures of exposure to individual smoke constituents as estimates of whole smoke exposure. The accuracy with which measurements of a single compound reflect exposure to whole smoke is limited by the changes in the composition of ETS with time and the conditions of exposure. For this reason, exposures to ETS are often assessed using several measures as markers, including markers of the vapor phase and the particulate phase as well as reactive and nonreactive constituents. Although biological markers show promise as measures of exposure because they measure the absorption of smoke constituents, they too have limitations. An individual's exposure is a dynamic integration of the concentration in various environments and the time that the individual spends in those environments.

In specifying an individual's exposure to specific components of ETS, consideration must be given to the time scale of exposure appropriate for the response of interest. Immediate exposures of seconds or hours would be most relevant for irritant and acute allergic responses. Time-averaged exposures, of hours or days, may be important for acute contemporary effects such as upper and lower respiratory tract symptoms or infections; chronic exposures occuring over a year or a lifetime might be associated with increased prevalence of chronic diseases and risk of cancer.

The spatial dimensions or the proximity of the individual to the source of smoke is important in assessing that individual's exposure to ETS. ETS is a complex, dynamic system that changes rapidly once emitted from a cigarette. Physical processes such as evaporation and dilution of the particles, scavenging of vapors on surfaces, and chemical reactions of reactive compounds are continuously occurring and modify the mixture referred to as ETS. An individual located a few centimeters or a meter from a burning cigarette may be exposed to a high concentration of ETS, ranging from 200 to 200 mg/m^3, and may inhale components of the mostly undiluted smoke plume and of the exhaled mainstream smoke. Studies have reported cigarette plume concentrations of formaldehyde and acrolein in the core smoke stream emitted from the cigarette of up to 100 times higher than known irritation levels. This "proximity effect" may be important in assessing exposure; distances on the order of a meter to tens of meters from a burning cigarette are relevant for exposures in offices, restaurants, home situations, automobiles, or the cabin of a commercial aircraft, because at these distances, the mixing of ETS throughout the airspace and the factors that affect concentration are important in determining exposure for people in that space. In many rooms, mixing is not completely uniform throughout the volume, and significant concentration gradients can be demonstrated. These gradients will affect an individual's exposure by modifying the effectiveness of ventilation in diluting or removing pollutants. The airborne mass concentration may vary by a factor of 10 or more within a room. Short-term measurements in rooms with smokers can yield respirable particulate components of 100 to 1,000 micrograms/m^3. Multihour measurements average out variations in smoking, mixing, and ventilation and yield concentrations in the range of 20 to 200 micrograms/m^3. Finally, on a systems scale, as in a house or building, concentrations are influenced by dispersion and dilution through the volume. Most time-integrated samples are taken on this larger scale.

Researchers have found significant variation in respirable suspended particulate levels between the living room, kitchen, and bedroom in homes during smoking or within one-half hour of smoking; others have noted, using tracer gases, that uniform concentrations are established in adjacent rooms within 30 to 90 minutes. Therefore, in a setting such as the work environment, where the duration of exposure is several hours or more, ETS would be expected to disseminate throughout the airspace in which smoking is occurring. Smoke dissemination may be reduced when air exchange rates are low, as may occur when internal doors are closed.

Time-Activity Patterns

Individual time-activity patterns are a major determinant of exposure to ETS. The population of the United States is mobile, spending variable amounts of time in different microenvironments. Individual activity patterns depend on age, occupation, season, social class, and sex. One study reported that in a certain community in Tennessee, the residents of the area spent 75% of their person-hours at home, 10.8% at work, 8.5% in public places, 2.9% in travel, and 2.8% in various other places. As expected, occupation and age were strong determinants of time-activity patterns in this study. Housewives and unemployed or retired persons spent 84.9% of their time at home, and occupational groups worked 21% to 24% of the hours. Students tended to spend the largest percentage of their time in public places, presumably schools, ranging from 14.7% for the youngest group to 19.17% for the oldest group of students.

A study, conducted in 1982, that contrasted various types of workers and the areas where they spent time (and whether they were near smokers) demonstrated that individual nonsmokers' exposure to smokers can be quite marked in various occupational groups.

Infants have unique time-activity patterns; their mobility is limited and the locations where they spend their time depends primarily on their caretakers. Although infants spend most of their time in their bedrooms, they are in contact with a caretaker while traveling, or in the living room, or kitchen for about half of the day. These time-activity patterns may also suggest that infants spending time in day-care may be exposed to ETS from smoking caretakers at commercial day-care centers, even though smoking may be restricted to special areas.

Although most people spend approximately 90% of their time in just two microenvironments (home and work), important exposures can be encountered in other environments. For example, commuting or being "in transit" accounts for about 0.5 to 1.5 hours each day for most persons; therefore, additional information on time spent and ETS concentrations in various microenvironments may be useful in defining exposure. The limitations in using this time-activity approach in characterizing exposures to various environmental pollutants, including ETS, are as follows: the extent to which overall population estimates can be generalized to individual patterns is poorly understood; concentrations in various microenvironments are only partially characterized; the variation in time and activity patterns and their effects on concentration levels are not established; extrapolation to longer time scales prospectively or retrospectively has not been validated; and the differences within structures, such as room to room variations, are not well established.

Temporal and Spatial Distribution of Smokers

Exposure to ETS can occur in a wide variety of public and private locations. Approximately 30% of the United States adult population currently are cigarette smokers. Nationwide, 40% of homes have one or more smokers (according to Bureau of Census figures). In surveys conducted in the past 10 years, the percentage of homes with smokers ranged from 54% to 75%. These data suggest that the population potentially exposed to ETS at home is greater than might be inferred from national statistics on the prevalence of smoking. However, the percentage of homes with smokers will vary among different regions, and smoking does not take place uniformly in time and space. Smoking patterns may change with activity, location, and time of day; all these variables serve to modify a nonsmoker's exposure to ETS.

Smoking prevalence varies widely among different groups; this variation modifies the exposure of nonsmokers to ETS. Smokers are present in nearly all environments, including most workplaces, restaurants, and transit vehicles, making it almost impossible for a nonsmoker to avoid some exposure to ETS. The number of cigarettes consumed per hour by the smoker may vary at different times of day, and the rate and density of smoking will also differ by the type of indoor environment and activity in such locales as schools, autos, planes, offices, shops, and bars.

Determinations of Concentration of Environmental Tobacco Smoke

ETS is a complex mixture of chemical compounds that individually may be in the particulate phase, the vapor phase, or both. ETS concentration varies with the generation rate of its tobacco-derived constituents, usually given as micrometer/hour. The generation rate for ETS has been approximated by the number of cigarettes smoked or the number of people present in a room who are actively smoking. Room-specific characteristics such as ventilation rate, decay rate, mixing rate, and room volume also modify the concentration. Because ETS particles have mass median diameters in the 0.2 to 0.4 micrometer range, convective flows dominate their movement in air, they remain airborne for long times, and they are rapidly distributed through a room by advection and other mixing forces. Under many conditions, the ventilation rate of a space will dominate chemical or physical removal mechanisms in determining levels of ETS particles.

Nonreactive ETS components distribute rapidly through an air-space volume, and their elimination depends almost solely on the ventilation rate. ETS-derived substances may decay as a function of the chemical and physical characteristics of room surfaces; carpet and furnishing types may change the removal characteristics of ETS.

Microenvironmental Measurements of Concentrations

The complex chemical makeup of ETS makes measurements of individual levels for each compound present in ETS impossible with existing resources; thus, some constituents have been measured as markers of overall smoke exposure. Because many of these constituents are also emitted from other sources in the environment, the contribution of ETS to the levels of these constituents is quantified by determining the enrichment of specific compounds found in smoke-polluted environments relative to the concentrations measured in nonsmoking areas. Various ETS components have been measured for this purpose, including acrolein, aldehydes, aromatic hydrocarbons, carbon monoxide, nicotine, nitrogen oxides, nitrosamines, phenols, and respirable particulate matter. The major limitation of using most of these substances is their lack of specificity for ETS. The presence of sources other than tobacco smoke for these compounds may limit their usefulness for determining the absolute contribution made by ETS to room concentrations. However, levels of nicotine and tobacco-specific nitrosamines are specific for ETS exposure.

A widely reported marker of ETS is respirable suspended particulate (RSP) matter; although lacking specificity for tobacco smoke, the prevalence and number of smokers correlates well with RSP levels in enclosed areas. Data on RSP levels in homes demonstrated that indoor concentrations were higher on the average and had a greater range than outdoor concentrations, therefore it can be seen that even one smoker can significantly elevate indoor RSP levels.

Researchers have found that the mean RSP concentration increased by 0.88 microgram/m^3 for every cigarette smoked per day; a one-pack per day smoker thus raises the indoor respirable particulate levels by 17.6 micrograms/m^3. Air conditioning increased the contribution of each cigarette by 1.23 micrograms/m^3, to a total of 2.11 micrograms/m^3 per cigarette in fully air conditioned areas. Air recirculation during summer months, when air conditioning is in place all day, will yield higher levels. Other studies utilizing measurements in large numbers of locations, using measures of smoke generation such as number of people smoking or the number of cigarettes smoked, have shown a definite relationship of smoke generation to particulate levels.

Nicotine appears to be a promising tracer for ETS because it is specific for tobacco and is present in relatively high concentrations in tobacco smoke. It can also be detected and measured in biological fluids to provide an indication of acute exposure to tobacco smoke. Cotinine, nicotine's major metabolite, can be used as an indicator of more chronic exposure. (These biological markers are discussed elsewhere in this book.) Recent studies have shown that nicotine may be primarily associated with the vapor phase of ETS and therefore, not a surrogate for the particulate phase as was once thought. However, the possible usefulness of this compound in estimating exposure to ETS warrants further evaluation. The nicotine content of sidestream smoke does not differ significantly from brand to brand when normalized on a per gram of tobacco basis. The use of nicotine as a marker for ETS must also take into account loss to surfaces and subsequent revolatilization and readmission to the room volume.

Carbon monoxide, a marker for gas phase components, has been measured extensively as a surrogate for ETS. There are many sources for carbon monoxide other than cigarettes in the indoor environment. This nonspecificity for ETS seriously limits its usefulness for environmental measurements.

Monitoring Studies

Personal monitors can measure the concentrations of ETS in a person's breathing zone. Personal monitoring is preferable to area monitoring because it integrates the temporal and spatial dimensions of an individual's exposure. Time-activity diaries have been found to permit greater resolution in attributing exposure to specific sources.

Personal monitoring techniques are currently available that will allow the assessment of individual exposures to various components of ETS. Although not widely used in the past, they can provide valuable input in developing exposure models and in validating other monitoring schemes. Their usefulness is primarily that they sample all the microenvironments in which individuals find themselves and therefore automatically compensate for nonuniform temporal and spatial distributions of ETS that affect personal exposure profiles.

HEALTH EFFECTS: INTRODUCTION

It is now accepted by most scientists, and endorsed by several Surgeons General of the United States, that cigarette and other tobacco smoking is the cause of most lung cancer and a substantial number of cancers at other sites, a large share of cardiovascular disease, and most chronic obstructive lung disease in the United States. The Office of Technology Assessment estimated that, in 1982, about 314,000 deaths in the United States were related to smoking, amounting to about 16% of all deaths in that year. The exact mechanisms by which tobacco smoking induces disease and the specific components of tobacco smoke that are harmful are not all known. It has been shown, however, that many of the individual constituents of tobacco smoke are carcinogenic in animals.

The mountain of evidence against tobacco smoking that has accumulated since the 1950s indicates that, among smokers, the level of health risk for the major effects increases with increasing dose. The age when a person starts smoking, the number of years of smoking, and the amount smoked per day all play a part in determining a smoker's risk of smoking-related disease or death. No level of smoking is thought to be "safe." This "dose-response" relationship, which is a commonly accepted tenet in assessing the effects of toxic chemicals, is one reason that investigations of possible health effects of passively inhaled smoke have been undertaken. Passive smoking results in much lower doses than smokers get, so nonsmokers' health risks, per person, should be smaller than the risks of smokers. The number of passively exposed individuals is larger than the number of smokers, however, so even at low levels of risk, a large number of people might be harmed through passive smoking. A particular concern of some investigators has been the possibility that some subgroups in the population, for instance children and those with preexisting lung disease or other chronic diseases, might be more sensitive to the effects of cigarette smoke than would be predicted from studies of smokers.

Much research has been directed at trying to characterize the risks from passive smoking, to determine whether they are or are not important public health concerns. Since the late 1970s, the pace of research on the health effects of passive smoking has increased considerably, and the body of literature now available is adequate, at least in some areas, to draw reasonable conclusions about the importance of passive smoking to the health of nonsmokers. Studies are not available to document many of the specific kinds of symptoms that people experience and report to physicians, such as various allergic reactions. Survey results support the fact that most smokers and nonsmokers are "annoyed" by tobacco smoke, annoyance undoubtedly taking in physical as well as psychological effects.

The health effects that have been investigated most extensively in relation to passive smoking in adults are lung cancer and alterations in lung function. There is a small literature concerning the relationship of passive smoking to cardiovascular symptoms and to death from ischemic heart disease. This topic has been discussed more fully in Chapter 1.

EXPOSURE TO ENVIRONMENTAL TOBACCO SMOKE: HEALTH EFFECTS

In 1964, the first Report of the Surgeon General on smoking and health determined that cigarette smoking was a cause of lung cancer, and noted causal relationships between smoking and other cancers, as well as chronic lung disease. Subsequent reports have noted association, both causal and noncausal, between tobacco smoking and a wide range of acute and chronic diseases. Epidemiological studies have documented the effects of tobacco smoking in humans; complementary laboratory studies have explained some of the mechanisms through which tobacco smoke causes disease.

More recently, the effects of inhalation of ETS by nonsmokers have become a pressing public health concern. Nonsmokers, as well as active smokers, inhale ETS, which is defined as the mixture of sidestream smoke and exhaled mainstream smoke. Various terms have been applied to the inhalation of ETS by nonsmokers; the terms "involuntary smoking" and "passive smoking" are the most prevalent and are often used interchangeably by researchers and the public.

Many of the known toxic and carcinogenic agents found in mainstream cigarette smoke have also been shown to be present in sidestream smoke. Furthermore, the combustion conditions under which sidestream smoke is produced result in the generation of larger amounts of many of these toxic and carcinogenic agents per gram of tobacco burned than the conditions under which mainstream smoke is generated. The characteristics of ETS also differ from those of mainstream smoke because the sidestream smoke ages before it is inhaled and the mainstream smoke exhaled by the active smoker is modified during its residence in the lung. There is no evidence to suggest that ETS has a qualitatively lower toxicity or carcinogenicity than mainstream smoke per milligram of smoke inhaled. In fact, the available evidence suggests that sidestream smoke contains higher concentrations of many known toxic and carcinogenic agents than mainstream smoke (according to animal tests). As a result, involuntary smoking should not be viewed as a qualitatively different exposure from active smoking, but rather as a low-dose exposure to a known hazardous agent, tobacco smoke.

Evaluation of Low-Dose Tobacco Smoke Exposure

Assessment of the health effects of any environmental exposure poses methodological problems, particularly when exposure levels are low and therefore the magnitude of the expected effect is small. The evaluation of an effect due to a low-dose exposure such as ETS requires the investigation of populations with differences in exposure large enough so that an effect could be anticipated. The population studied must also be of sufficient size to quantitate the effects in the range of interest with precision. Failure to fulfill these requirements may produce a false-negative result in a study of low-dose exposure.

Exposure to ETS is a nearly universal experience in the more developed countries, so the identification of a truly unexposed population is very difficult. Sample size considerations are also of particular concern for the epidemiological studies of lung cancer and involuntary smoking. Given the constraints of sample size and the varying gradients of exposure, it would be expected that some studies would find no association between involuntary smoking and lung cancer, and others studies would find associations that lacked statistical significance. Nonuniformity of data does not imply lack of effect; rather, it is the coherence and trends of the evidence that must be examined.

In evaluating the hazards posed by an air pollutant such as ETS, laboratory, toxicological, human exposure, and epidemiological investigations provide relevant data. Each approach has limitations, but the insights each provides are complementary. Epidemiology describes the effects in human populations, but results must be interpreted in the context of other forms of study.

Risk assessment techniques have also been used to characterize the potential adverse health effects of human exposures to environmental pollutants, particularly those at low levels. The four steps of risk assessment have been described by the National Academy of Sciences as hazard identification, dose-response assessment, exposure assessment, and risk characterization. Risk assessment has also been used to describe the consequences of exposure to ETS. However, unlike many environmental exposures for which risk assessment represents the only approach for estimating human risk, the health effects of ETS exposure can be directly examined using epidemiological methods. Conclusions presented in this document are based on laboratory, toxicological, and epidemiological evidence.

In the following pages, the literature on lung cancer, chronic obstructive lung disease, cardiovascular disease, and irritation is reviewed.

Lung Cancer and Passive Smoking

The first major studies linking passive smoking to lung cancer were published in 1981. Since then, about a dozen other studies, of various designs and in different parts of the world, have been completed, and the first two studies have been updated. The study populations are made up mainly, though not exclusively, of women. Studies that have a significant focus on passive smoking and lung cancer have been carried out in Hong Kong, Germany, and in different parts of the United States. Epidemiologic study of lung cancer and passive smoking continues, with at least two other studies nearing publication, and a heightening of interest among researchers.

In the United States, an estimated 9000 to 11,000 nonsmokers die of lung cancer each year, out of a total of about 100,000 lung cancer deaths. About one-third of the nonsmokers who die of lung cancer are men and two-thirds are women. The percentages of different cancer types (mainly adenocarcinomas and squamous cell carcinomas) differ between smokers and nonsmokers, suggesting at least some different causes in nonsmokers. Passive smoking may account for a portion of these deaths among nonsmokers, but there also are other as yet unknown causes.

Most of the studies have reported results consistent with approximately a doubling in the risk of lung cancer among nonsmokers heavily exposed to environmental tobacco smoke compared with nonsmokers who were not regularly exposed; some studies report larger increased risks, some smaller, and two studies found no increase. Passive smoking exposure may vary considerably around the world because of social customs and living conditions, so it is not unreasonable to expect risks to differ among studies. In five studies, statistically significant increased risks are reported.

The International Agency for Research on Cancer (IARC), a unit of the World Health Organization, reviewed some of the published studies as part of a monograph about the carcinogenic effects of smoking; the monograph was published in 1988. IARC notes that the risk estimates could actually be somewhat higher or lower than were calculated because of the uncertainties in measurements of passive exposure to cigarette smoke, as well as to other exposures that might have contributed to the development of lung cancer. Because the results could have been influenced by these uncertainties, IARC concludes that each study is compatible with either an increase or an absence of excess risk of lung cancer from passive exposure to tobacco smoke, even though statistically significant results were reported.

A recent case-control study, published in 1985, reported the passive smoking histories of 134 nonsmoking women with lung cancer as compared with the passive smoking histories of 402 nonsmoking women with colon-rectum cancer (cancers not known to be associated with smoking). Information was collected about several different aspects of passive exposure to cigarette smoke: current smoking habits of husbands or other cohabitants; number of cigarettes smoked per day at home by the cohabitant smokers; number of years the cohabitant smoked; average number of hours per day the women had been exposed to smoke of others during the past 5 and 25 years at home, at work, or elsewhere, and during childhood.

Data were analyzed using a variety of standard statistical methods. In almost all cases, the women with lung cancer were somewhat more likely to have been passively exposed to cigarette smoke than were the controls (the women with colo-rectal cancers). Most of the differences were not statistically significant, meaning that, using generally accepted statistical standards, the results could be plausible explained by chance alone. Several comparisons, however, did produce statistically significant results. For those results, chance alone is an unlikely explanation of the findings.

The strongest evidence for an effect of passive smoking in this study is from an analysis of risk related to the number of cigarettes smoked by the cohabitant per day in total, and the number smoked at home. The risks for women whose cohabitants smoked more that 40 cigarettes per day (two packs) total, or more than 20 cigarettes per day (one pack) at home were significantly higher than the risks for women whose cohabitants did not smoke. More importantly, there was a trend of increasing risk that rose significantly with higher categories of cohabitant's daily cigarette consumption.

As expected, the level of increased risk is much lower than the substantial increase in the risk of lung cancer incurred by smokers. Lifetime smokers are on the order of 10 to 15 times more likely to develop lung cancer than are lifetime nonsmokers. Data indicate that the risk of lung cancer among women passively exposed to the smoke of 20 cigarettes per day, smoked at home by cohabitants, is somewhat greater than two times the risk of nonsmoking women not passively exposed to cigarette smoke.

All the lung cancer studies have some methodologic weaknesses, and these have been pointed out; a small number of the studies include so few lung cancers or have such major flaws that they are essentially disregarded in this summary of the literature. The studies that can be evaluated vary greatly in design and the poplations studied vary, yet the results are generally consistent with an increased risk of lung cancer from passive smoking, even taking into account those weaknesses. This consistence across studies lends weight to an overall evaluation that no single study can achieve.

Effects of Passive Smoking on Lung Function

The 1984 Surgeon General's report examined the relationship of direct smoking to chronic obstructive lung disease, which killed more than 66,000 Americans in 1983. The report stated that the experimental and epidemiologic evidence left no room for reasonable doubt on the fundamental issue that cigarette smoking is the major cause of this type of lung disease in the United States. The report also reviewed the studies of the relationship between passive smoking and chronic obstructive lung disease and lung function published to that time. The information presented here is taken largely from the Surgeon General's report and other critical reviews of the literature on the health effects of passive smoking.

In general, chronic obstructive lung disease refers to the narrowing of the airways of the bronchial tree and loss of elasticity of the lungs, with a resultant loss of airflow driving pressure. Increased secretion of mucous and an increase in the size of mucous glands, as well as inflammation, abnormal cell types, ulceration, and a variety of other changes in the cellular makeup and condition of lung and bronchial tissue are also signs of chronic obstructive lung disease. Emphysema, characterized by specific pathologic changes in lung tissue, is the type of chronic lung disease most closely associated with smoking. While most diagnoses of chronic lung disease are in middle-aged or older people, a diagnosis is preceded by pathologic changes and measurable declines in lung function, which may occur over a period of decades.

The pertinent questions in regard to passive smoking are whether passive smoking contributes to the development of chronic obstructive lung disease, and whether passive smoking exacerbates the symptoms of, or has long-term adverse effects on, people with preexisting chronic obstructive lung disease.

The studies performed in this area were basically laboratory-based experiments in controlled chambers, in which the endpoints were short-term changes in lung function, and epidemiologic studies of the relationship between passive exposure to cigarette smoke and either measures of lung function or morbidity. Most of the epidemiologic studies focus on children, classified according to parental smoking. Investigators have studied the exposure of healthy people, to find out whether those passively exposed to tobacco smoke are more likely to develop respiratory problems than those not exposed; and those with respiratory conditions, particularly asthma, to see whether exposure exacerbates those conditions.

The Office of Technology Assessment, in its review, concentrated on studies of adults, the main targets of workplace smoking policies. However, children may be passively exposed to tobacco smoke in federal offices, for example, in agencies where federal workers deal directly with the public. In addition, at least a portion of the adult population may be as sensitive as children to the effects of passive smoking. Other reviewers have evaluated the evidence for respiratory system effects of passive smoking in children. One researcher reported that several studies had suggested important increases in severe respiratory illnesses in very young (less than 2 years old) children of smoking parents. Also cited was evidence of respiratory symptoms in older children exposed to environmental tobacco smoke. The evidence linking passive smoking with acute respiratory illnesses, chronic respiratory symptoms, and mild impairments of pulmonary function in children is strong.

Experimental Studies of Healthy Subjects

A few investigations have been conducted on subjects exposed to tobacco smoke in laboratory chambers with controlled atmospheres; measurements of lung function and, in some cases, measurements of carboxyhemoglobin levels were carried out at specific times during the experiment. The pulmonary function tests used in these experiments consist largely of measuring the volume of air that is moved in and out of the lungs under different conditions. Two of three such studies noted by the Surgeon General reported measurable decreases from initial levels in some measures of lung function after exposure of health volunteers to tobacco smoke. In another study which included both healthy volunteers and asthmatics, no statistically significant change in lung function after exposure to environmental tobacco smoke was found in the healthy subjects.

Epidemiologic Studies of Healthy Adults

Studies of pulmonary function in healthy adults, classified as to their passive smoking history, were reported in the Surgeon

General's 1984 report. Some of the studies found no effect on pulmonary function as a function of spouses' smoking status; however, the study populations were relatively young and might not have had long-term passive exposure to cigarette smoke.

Other studies have reported statistically significant, small losses in pulmonary function related to passive smoking. In one study, tobacco smoke at work was used as the measure of exposure, so it was really a study of current exposure, not necessarily representative of long-term exposure. Another study was made of nonsmoking women married to smokers; the women had lower values for one measure of pulmonary function than did similar women married to nonsmokers, but the effect did not become apparent until the women had reached age 40. The findings are not ascribable to differences in social class, educational status, exposure to air pollution, or family size.

Studies of Adults With Asthma

Studies of asthmatic adults, conducted in controlled environmental chambers, are reported by the Surgeon General; 10 patients with asthma and 10 healthy controls were exposed to environmental tobacco smoke. Similar increases in blood carboxyhemoglobin levels were found in both groups. The asthmatics, however, experienced worsening pulmonary function over the course of the one-hour experiment, while no change was detected among the controls. Another study on pulmonary function bore out this effect; the asthmatic group reported an increase in wheezing and chest tightness.

A recent study of 9 asthmatics, with normal or nearly normal lung function who were asymptomatic at the time of the test, found no significant change in lung function tests after 1 hour of tobacco smoke exposure in an experimental chamber. In addition to lung function tests, the investigators performed a test to determine whether tobacco smoke exposure increased the reactivity of the subjects' lungs when exposed to a chemical that causes an airway reaction. A high degree of reactivity is characteristic of asthmatics. After exposure to environmental tobacco smoke, the asthmatics were slightly less sensitive to the chemical than they had been before exposure, though they were still more sensitive than were a group of nonasthmatics.

Summary: Effects on Lung Function

There is currently a small literature on the effects of passive smoking on lung function in healthy adults, although there are no longitudinal studies. The experimental studies used a variety of tests and selected participants in different ways, some based on self-assessment of adverse effects of passive smoking. There is significant heterogeneity among the total population with some form of chronic obstructive lung disease, and the experimental studies that have been done examined small, selected groups that may not have represented average or most sensitive individuals in that population. It is difficult, therefore, to generalize from these results to the total population.

The assessment of effects of passive smoking on lung function and disease in healthy and compromised individuals would benefit greatly from further research. However, the studies to date do suggest a small acute effect of passive smoking on lung function in healthy adults; a 1983 study suggests a long-term adverse effect. The studies relating passive smoking to acute effects in adult asthmatics are at variance. There appears to be insufficient evidence to make conclusions about acute effects of passive smoking on patients with asthma or chronic obstructive lung disease, but it is likely that some proportion of these persons will be adversely affected.

PASSIVE SMOKING AND CARDIOVASCULAR DISEASE

Smoking is estimated to have contributed to 123,000 deaths from cardiovascular disease in the United States in 1982. This strong relationship underlies much of the concern about the potential for passive smoking to increase the cardiovascular disease risk of nonsmokers.

Epidemiologic Studies

Researchers in Scotland found no association of cardiovascular conditions with passive smoking in men or women; a Japanese researcher found small, statistically significant, increases in the risk of death from ischemic heart disease among wives of smokers and ex-smokers. In a study done in the United States, an increased risk of death from ischemic heart disease among wives of current or former smokers was found, but the result was not statistically significant.

Experimental Studies

The focus of experimental studies has been to determine the effect of acute exposure to carbon monoxide and environmental tobacco smoke on patients with angina. The literature is summarized in the 1979 Surgeon General's *Report on Smoking and Health*. These studies showed that, after exposure to environmental tobacco smoke, angina pain began sooner than it did in the absence of exposure. While there is agreement that an increase of about 5% in carboxyhemoglobin levels can measurably shorten the time to onset of anginal pain, there is still insufficient evidence to determine whether an increase in carboxyhemoglobin caused by passive smoking, which has been measured in the range of 2–3%, can be sufficient to produce an effect.

Summary: Cardiovascular Effects

The available epidemiologic data point to an increased risk of death from ischemic heart disease among nonsmokers exposed to environmental tobacco smoke, but there are too few studies to make final judgments. The experimental evidence suggests that patients with ischemic heart disease could suffer a worsening of symptoms with exposure to environmental tobacco smoke.

IRRITATION

The most widespread acute physical effects of passive exposure to cigarette smoke are various types of "irritation." Eye irritation is the commonest complaint, but headaches, coughs, and irritation of the nose are also commonly reported. In one study cited in the 1984 Surgeon General's report, 69% of subjects reported eye irritation at some time in response to cigarette smoke. In one experimental chamber study, both a subjective and an objective measure of eye irritation were recorded. After an hour of exposure at smoke levels similar to those found in many public places, including offices, study participants reported increased eye irritation, and the objective measure, the rate of eye blinking, also increased. Annoying and irritating effects of passive cigarette smoke exposure increases with smoke concentration. A tolerable limit of passive smoke exposure that lies in the range between 1.5 and 2.0 ppm carbon monoxide, is suggested.[10] Eye irritation is also reported incidentally in various experimental studies of passive smoking. In a 1986 experimental study of adult asthmatics reported in the Office of Technology Assessment Study,[11] the authors noted that marked eye irritation was a universal finding, and that nasopharyngeal irritation was also common. After several minutes in the experimental chamber, most subjects chose to wear goggles offered to protect their eyes from smoke.

There is sufficient evidence from surveys and observational studies that most people, including many smokers, are physically irritated by tobacco smoke. The means to test this belief is limited, and few studies have done so, but the effect is generally accepted.

Health Effects: Summary

Taken individually, much of the evidence for adverse health effects related to passive smoking is equivocal. As is the case for nearly every other body of health effects literature, there are few "definitive" studies that by themselves change scientific thinking. Conclusions are drawn by examining the aggregate of studies and weighing their designs, flaws, and findings. In the case of passive smoking, the available evidence taken together supports stronger conclusions than do the individual studies.

Studies of respiratory effects suggest that people with asthma can be harmed by environmental tobacco smoke. Healthy adults may experience measurable disturbances of pulmonary function from passive smoke exposure. There is evidence that environmental tobacco smoke is an acute respiratory irritant, and an eye irritant. While the acute, short-term effects of passive smoking are by themselves relevant for a study of workplace smoking policies, their long-term health implications are less clear.

Evidence linking passive smoking to cardiovascular disease and symptoms is still rather scanty, but some studies suggest both acute exacerbation of angina pain and an increased risk of death from heart disease. The plausibility of these conclusions is supported by the known cardiovascular effects of direct smoking.

The epidemiologic evidence from a number of studies is generally consistent with the biologically plausible hypothesis that passive exposure to tobacco smoke can cause lung cancer. Taken together, the evidence points to a carcinogenic effect smaller than that observed for direct cigarette smoking. The published studies to date have not been free of flaws in methodology and design, particularly in their measurement of the extent of subjects' exposure to environmental tobacco smoke, but these flaws do not invalidate the studies. Even the best of such studies have not achieved the methodological precision of studies of direct smoking and lung cancer. Still, because so many people are currently exposed to environmental tobacco smoke, even a small increase in the risk of lung cancer from passive smoking would be important. Despite the uncertainties in the evidence, the data are sufficient to warrant serious concern.

EXPOSURE TO ENVIRONMENTAL TOBACCO SMOKE: OCCUPATIONAL CONSIDERATIONS

Cigarette smoking may influence the effects of hazardous occupational inhalants. It seems clear that smoking is an important factor, perhaps as a cocarcinogen, in the induction of most occupational lung cancers.[12] Elimination of smoking in certain occupational settings would significantly reduce the occurrence of disease in the workplace.[13,14]

Chronic Bronchitis: Interaction of Smoking and Occupation

Chronic simple bronchitis has been associated with occupational exposures in both nonsmoking exposed workers and populations of exposed smokers in excess of rates predicted from the smoking habit alone. Among these exposures are coal, grain, silica, the welding environment, and to a lesser extent, sulfur dioxide and cement. The evidence indicated that the effects of smoking and those occupational agents that cause bronchitis are frequently additive in producing symptoms of chronic cough and expectoration. Smoking has commonly been demonstrated to be the more important factor in producing these symptoms.

Asbestos-Exposed Workers

Asbestos exposure can increase the risk of developing lung cancer in both cigarette smokers and nonsmokers. The risk in cigarette-smoking asbestos workers is greater than the sum of the risks of the independent exposures, and is approximated by multiplying the risks of the separate exposures. The risk of developing lung cancer in asbestos workers increases with increasing number of cigarettes smoked per day and increasing cumulative asbestos exposure.[15] Employment in asbestos insulation work greatly increases the lung cancer risk of cigarette smokers, and may increase their risk of asbestosis.[16]

The risk of developing lung cancer declines in asbestos workers who stop smoking when compared with asbestos workers who continue to smoke. Cessation of asbestos exposure may result in a lower risk of developing lung cancer than continued exposure, but the risk of developing lung cancer appears to remain significantly elevated even after 25 years after cessation of exposure.[17]

Cigarette smoking and asbestos exposure appear to have an independent and additive effect on lung function decline. Nonsmoking asbestos workers have decreased total lung capacities (restrictive disease). Cigarette-smoking asbestos workers develop both restrictive lung disease and chronic obstructive lung disease, but the evidence does not suggest that cigarette-smoking asbestos workers have a lower lung capacity as measured by spirometry than would be expected from their smoking habits alone.[18,19,20]

Both cigarette smoking and asbestos exposure result in an increased resistance to airflow in the small airways. In the absence of cigarette smoking, this increased resistance in the small airways does not appear to result in obstruction on standard spirometric tests. Asbestos exposure is the predominant cause of interstitial fibrosis in populations with substantial asbestos exposure. Cigarette smokers do have a slightly higher prevalence of chest radiographs interpreted as interstitial fibrosis than nonsmokers, but neither the frequency of these changes nor the severity of the changes approach levels found in populations with substantial asbestos exposure.[21,22,23,24]

The promotion of smoking cessation should be an intrinsic part of efforts to control asbestos-related death and disability.[25]

Respiratory Disease in Coal Miners

Coal dust exposure is clearly the major etiological factor in the production of the radiologic changes of coal workers' pneumoconiosis (CWP). Cigarette smoking probably increases the prevalence of irregular opacities on the chest x-rays of smoking coal miners, but appears to have little effect on the prevalence of small rounded opacities or complicated CWP. Increasing severity categories of simple radiologic CWP are not associated with increasing airflow obstruction, but increasing coal dust exposure is associated with increasing airflow obstruction in both smokers and nonsmokers.

Since the introduction of more effective controls to reduce the level of coal dust exposure at the worksite, cigarette smoking has become the more significant contributor to reported cases of disabling airflow obstruction among coal miners. Cigarette smoking and coal dust exposure appear to have an independent and additive effect on the prevalence of chronic cough and phlegm. Increasing coal dust exposure is associated with a form of emphysema known as focal dust emphysema, but there is no definite evidence that extensive centrilobular emphysema occurs in the absence of cigarette smoking. The majority of studies have shown that coal dust exposure is not associated with an increased risk for lung cancer.

Reduction in the levels of coal dust exposure is the only method available to reduce the prevalence of simple or complicated CWP. However, the prevalence of ventilatory disabilities in coal miners could be substantially reduced by reducing the prevalence of cigarette smoking, and efforts aimed at reducing ventilatory disability should include efforts to enhance successful smoking cessation.

Silica-Exposed Workers

Silicosis, acute silicosis, mixed-dust silicosis, silicotuberculosis, and diatomaceous earth pneumoconiosis are causally related to silica exposure as a sole or principal etiological agent. Epidemiological evidence, based on both cross-sectional and prospective studies, demonstrates that silica dust is associated with chronic bronchitis and chronic airways obstruction. Silica dust and smoking are major risk factors and appear to be additive in producing chronic bronchitis and chronic airways obstruction. Most studies indicate that the smoking effect is stronger than the silica dust effect.

Pathology studies describe mineral dust airways disease, which is morphologically similar to the small airways lesions caused by cigarette smoking. A number of studies have demonstrated an increased risk of lung cancer in workers exposed to silica, but few of these studies have been adequately controlled for smoking. Therefore, while the increased standardized mortality rates for lung cancer in these populations suggest the need for further investigation of a potential carcinogenic effect of silica exposure (particularly in a combined exposure with other possible carcinogens), the evidence does not currently establish whether silica exposure increases the risk of developing lung cancer in man.

Smoking control efforts should be an important concomitant of efforts to reduce the burden of silica related illness in working populations.

Workers Exposed to Grain Dust

Cumulative smoking and respirable dust concentration adversely affect pulmonary function by impairing the small airways.[26] Smoking delays the clearance of dust from the airways of grain workers.[27] As is the case with other dust involved lung diseases, specific dust exposure, advancing age, and tobacco smoking contribute to the pathogenesis of chronic airflow irritation.[28]

Occupational Exposures to Petrochemicals, Aromatic Amines, and Pesticides

The biotransformation of industrial toxicants can be modified, at least to some extent, by the constituents of tobacco smoke through enzyme induction or possibly inhibition. Both tobacco smoke and some industrial pollutants contain substances capable of initiating and promoting cancer and damaging the airways and lung parenchyma. There is, therefore, an ample biologic basis for suspecting that important interactive effects exist between some workplace pollutants and tobacco smoke.

In mortality studies of coke oven workers and gas workers, convincing evidence has indicated that work exposures to oven effluents cause an excess risk of lung cancer in spite of the lack of adequate information on smoking. Other mortality studies that suggest small increases in smoking related diseases, such as pancreatic cancer in refinery workers, cannot be interpreted without more information on smoking. For bladder cancer, the interactions between smoking and occupational exposure are unclear, with both additive and antagonistic interactions having been demonstrated. Relative risk of bladder cancer was 1.5 and 1.9 for men who had never smoked and men who were current smokers respectively. Increased risk for cancer was associated with greater levels of smoking. Those with the greatest relative risks for bladder cancer were janitors and cleaners, mechanics, mining machine operators, and printing machine operators. Workers in metal mining industries had the greatest risk of bladder cancer. Other high risk groups included plumbers, metal machinists, and truck drivers.[29,30,31] The risk of pulmonary disability in rubber workers was increased when smoking and occupational exposure to particulates were combined. There are few empirical animal experiments for lung disease that demonstrate interactive effects between cigarette smoking and various industrial chemicals.

Workers involved in the manufacture of polymeric materials have experienced disease as a consequence of their exposure to the cofactors of petrochemicals and smoking. Workers who smoke transfer fluorocarbon polymers to cigarettes from their hands, allowing the subsequent production of pyrolysis products while smoking; this, results in the contraction of polymer fume fever.[32,33] Both styrene exposure and smoking are damaging to cytogenetic and cytokinetic aspects of lymphocytes.[34,35]

Cotton Dust Exposure and Cigarette Smoking

Byssinosis prevalence and severity is increased in cotton textile workers who smoke, in comparison with workers who do not smoke. Cigarette smoking seems to facilitate byssinosis in workers exposed to cotton dust, perhaps by the prior induction of bronchitis. Cotton mill workers of both sexes who smoke have a consistently greater prevalence of bronchitis than nonsmokers. The importance of cigarette smoking to byssinosis prevalence seems to grow with rising dust levels (a smoking-cotton interaction). At the highest dust levels, cigarette smoke was found to interact with cotton dust exposure to substantially increase the prevalence of acute symptoms.[36]

Nonsmokers with byssinosis have lower preshift lung function and a greater cross-shift decline in lung function than asymptomatic workers, and those workers with bronchitis generally have lower preshift lung function than those without bronchitis. In general, smokers have lower lung function than nonsmokers among cotton workers, both in those with bronchitis and in those with byssinosis. Although the average forced expiration values measured at the start of a shift are reduced in smokers, the cross-shift decline in function does not seem to be affected by smoking status.

The contribution of the acute byssinotic symptoms to the subsequent development of what have been termed the chronic forms of byssinosis (which include airways obstruction) is not well documented; however, chronic airflow obstruction has been found more frequently in cotton textile workers than in control populations, and this lung function loss appears to be additive to that caused by cigarette smoking. Cotton dust exposure is significantly associated with mucous gland volume and peripheral goblet cell metaplasia in nonsmokers, a pathology consistent with bronchitis. In cigarette smokers, the interaction of cotton textile exposure and smoking is demonstrable for goblet cell hyperplasia. Centrilobular emphysema is found only in association with cigarette smoking and pipe smoking. There is no emphysema association found with cotton dust exposure. The evidence does not currently suggest an excess risk of lung cancer among cotton textile workers. However, pulmonary function in cotton workers tends to improve in nonsmokers and former smokers only upon continued nonsmoking. Chronic obstructive pulmonary disease may not be reversible even among retired cotton workers.[37]

Ionizing Radiation and Lung Cancer

There is an interaction between radon daughters and cigarette smoke exposures in the production of lung cancer in both man and animals. The nature of this interaction is not entirely clear because of the conflicting results in both epidemiological and animal studies. The interaction between radon daughters and cigarette smoke exposures may consist of two parts. The first is an additive effect on the number of cancers induced by the two agents; the second is the hastening effect of the tumor promoters in cigarette smoke on the appearance of cancers induced by radiation, so that the induction latent period is shorter among smokers than among nonsmokers, and the resultant cancers are distributed in time differently between smokers and nonsmokers, appearing earlier in smokers. Uranium miners, exposed to radioactive minerals during the course of their employment, may run higher risks for cancer if they are smokers.[38] There appears to be a synergistic effect between smoking and radon radiation in lung cancer.[39,40] Because smoking alone cannot explain the marked excess of lung cancer in uranium miners, and because smoking differences cannot account for the increasing cancer risks in relation to increased radiation exposure, uranium miners should not smoke.[41]

REFERENCES

1. Husgafvel-Pursiainen, K., M. Sorsa, K. Engstrom, and P. Einisto. ''Passive smoking at work: Biochemical and biological measures of exposure to environmental tobacco smoke.'' *International Archives of Occupational and Environmental Health* 59(4), 337–345, 1987. (NIOSH-00175679)

2. Lee, H.K., T.A. McKenna, L.N. Renton, and J. Kirkbride. "Impact of a new smoking policy on office air quality," *Indoor Air Quality in Cold Climates: Hazards and Abatement Measures,* edited by D.S. Walkinshaw. Pittsburgh, PA: Air Pollution Control Association, 1986. pp. 307–322. (NIOSH-00172085)

3. Jarvis, M.J., M.A.H. Russell, and C. Feyerabend. "Absorption of nicotine and carbon monoxide from passive smoking under natural conditions of exposure," *Thorax* 38(11), 829–833, 1983. (NIOSH-00144535)

4. *Health Consequences of Involuntary Smoking: A Report of the Surgeon General.* U.S. Department of Health and Human Services, Public Health Service. Washington, DC: Superintendent of Documents, U.S. Government Printing Office, 1986. 359 pp. DHHS(CDC)87-8398. pp. 7, 21–28, 132–147, 164–169, 181–198, 229–252, 265–308.

5. Lewis, G.P., W.J. Jusko, and L.L. Coughlin. "Cadmium accumulation in man: Influence of smoking, occupation, alcoholic habit and disease," *Journal of Chronic Diseases* 25(12), 717–726, 1972. (NIOSH-00155643)

6. Pukkala, E., L. Teppo, T. Hakulinen, and M. Rimpela. "Occupation and smoking as risk determinants of lung cancer," *International Journal of Epidemiology* 12(3), 290–296, 1983. (NIOSH-00147178)

7. Pershagen, G., S. Wall, A. Taube, and L. Linnman. "On the interaction between occupational arsenic exposure and smoking and its relationship to lung cancer," *Scandinavian Journal of Work, Environment and Health* 7(4), 302–309, 1981. (NIOSH-00157745)

8. Siegers, C.P., J.R. Jungblut, F. Klink, and F. Oberheuser. "Effect of smoking on cadmium and lead concentrations in human amniotic fluid," *Toxicology Letters* 19(3), 327–331, 1983. (NIOSH-00139819)

9. Blanusa, M., Z. Kralj, and A. Bunarevic. "Interaction of cadmium, zinc and copper in relation to smoking habit, age and histopathological findings in human kidney cortex," *Archives of Toxicology* 58(4), 115–117, 1985. (NIOSH-00159033)

10. Muramatsu, T., A. Weber, S. Muramatsu, and F. Akermann. "An experimental study on irritation and annoyance due to passive smoking," *International Archives of Occupational and Environmental Health* 51(4), 305–317, 1983. (NIOSH-00144350)

11. *Passive Smoking in the Workplace: Selected Issues*. Staff paper prepared by the Special Projects Office of the Health Program, Office of Technology Assessment: U.S. Congress, 1986. 70 pp. (NTIS PB86-217627). pp. 1–2, 4–5, 8–59.

12. Weill, H., and J. Diem. "Relationships between cigarette smoking and occupational pulmonary disease," *Occupational Pulmonary Disease: Focus on Grain Dust and Health,* edited by J.A. Dosman and D.J. Cotton. NY: Academic Press, 1977. pp. 65–75. (NIOSH-00158415)

13. Kotin, P., and L.A. Gaul. "Smoking in the workplace: A hazard ignored," *American Journal of Public Health* 70(6), 575–576, 1980. (NIOSH-00130536)

14. Chovill, A.C. "Occupational lung cancer and smoking: A review in the light of current theories of carcinogenesis," *Canadian Medical Association Journal* 121, 548–555, Sept. 8, 1979. (NIOSH-00133839)

15. Grimson, R.C. "Apportionment of risk among environmental exposures: Application to asbestos exposure and cigarette smoking," *Journal of Occupational Medicine* 29(3), 253–255, 1987. (NIOSH-00167847)

16. Hammond, E.C., and I.J. Selikoff. "Relation of cigarette smoking to risk of death of asbestos-associated disease among insulation workers in the United States," *Biological Effects of Asbestos* (IARC Scientific Publication No. 8), pp. 312–317, 1973. (NIOSH-00149797)

17. Hilt, B., S. Langard, A. Andersen, and J. Rosenberg. "Asbestos exposure, smoking habits, and cancer incidence among production and maintenance workers in an electrochemical plant," *American Journal of Industrial Medicine* 8(6), 565–577, 1985. (NIOSH-00136894)

18. Richter, E.D., H. Tuch, O. Sarel, Z. Shabbat, and D. Weiler. "Smoking, morbidity, and pulmonary function in a group of ex-asbestos workers: A pilot study," *American Journal of Industrial Medicine* 10(5/6), 515–523, 1986. (NIOSH-00164999)

19. Saracci, R. "Asbestos and lung cancer: An analysis of the epidemiological evidence on the asbestos-smoking interaction," *International Journal of Cancer* 20(3), 323–331, 1977. (NIOSH-00073561)

20. Miller, A., J.C. Thornton, R. Warshaw, A.S. Teirstein, and I.J. Selikoff. "Pulmonary function in two asbestos-exposed occupational groups: Comparison with a reference population by smoking history," *European Journal of Respiratory Diseases* 62(113), 1–2, 1982. (NIOSH-00126893)

21. Begin, R., R. Boileau, and S. Peloquin. "Asbestos exposure, cigarette smoking, and airflow limitation in long-term Canadian chrysotile miners and millers," *American Journal of Industrial Medicine* 11(1), 55–66, 1987. (NIOSH-00166361)

22. Kjuus, H., R. Skjaerven, S. Langard, J.T. Lien, and T. Aamodt. "A case-referent study of lung cancer, occupational exposures and smoking. II. Role of asbestos exposure," *Scandinavian Journal of Work, Environment and Health* 12(3), 203–209, 1986. (NIOSH-00163440)

23. Sue, D.Y., A. Oren, J.E. Hansen, and K. Wasserman. "Lung function and exercise performance in smoking and nonsmoking asbestos-exposed workers," *American Review of Respiratory Disease* 132(3), 612–618, 1985. (NIOSH-00154050)

24. Pearle, J.L. "Smoking and duration of asbestos exposure in the production of functional and roentgenographic abnormalities in shipyard workers," *Journal of Occupational Medicine* 24(1), 37–40, 1982. (NIOSH-00121566)

25. Selikoff, I.J., E.C. Hammond, and J. Churg. "Asbestos exposure, smoking, and neoplasia," *Journal of the American Medical Association* 204(2), 106–112, Apr. 8, 1968. (NIOSH-00127939)

26. Carta, P., P.L. Cocco, G. Aru, M.T. Barbieri, E. Cocco, M. Meloni, F. Sanna-Randaccio, and D. Casula. "Smoking and dust effects upon lung function of healthy workers," *European Journal of Respiratory Diseases* 62(113), 26–27, 1982. (NIOSH-00126900)

27. Dosman, J.A. "Chronic obstructive pulmonary disease and smoking in grain workers," *Occupational Pulmonary Disease: Focus on Grain Dust and Health,* edited by J.A. Dosman and D.J. Cotton. NY: Academic Press, 1980. pp. 201–206. (NIOSH-00157351)

28. Bachani, D. "Chronic airflow limitation in talc industry: Role of age, smoking habits and dust exposure," *Indian Journal of Chest Diseases and Allied Sciences* 26(4), 220–224, 1984. (NIOSH-00161671)

29. Brownson, R.C., J.C. Chang, and J.R. Davis. "Occupation, smoking, and alcohol in the epidemiology of bladder cancer," *American Journal of Public Health* 77(10), 1298–1300, 1987. (NIOSH-00173444)

30. Vineis, P., N. Segnan, G. Costa, and B. Terracini. "Evidence of a multiplicative effect between cigarette smoking and occupational exposures in the aetiology of bladder cancer," *Cancer Letter* 14(3), 285–290, 1981. (NIOSH-00120374)

31. Cartwright, R. "Occupational bladder cancer and cigarette smoking in West Yorkshire," *Scandinavian Journal of Work, Environment and Health* 8(1), 79–82, 1982. (NIOSH-00125060)

32. Wegman, D.H., and J.M. Peters, "Polymer fume fever and cigarette smoking," *Annals of Internal Medicine* 81(1), 55–57, 1974. (NIOSH-00128434)

33. Welti, D.W., and M.J. Hipp. "Polymer fume fever. Possible relationship to smoking," *Journal of Occupational Medicine* 10(11), 667–671, 1968. (NIOSH-00128869)

34. Watanabe, T., A. Endo, M. Kumai, and M. Ikeda. "Chromosome aberrations and sister chromatid exchanges in styrene-exposed workers with reference to their smoking habits," *Environmental Mutagenesis* 5(3), 299–309, 1983. (NIOSH-00138347)

35. Albrecht, W.N., and C.J. Bryant. "Polymer-fume fever associated with smoking and use of a mold-release spray containing polytetrafluoroethylene," *Journal of Occupational Medicine* 29(10), 817–819, 1987. (NIOSH-00174913)

36. Beck, G.J., L.R. Maunder, and E.N. Schachter. "Cotton dust and smoking effects on lung function in cotton textile workers," *American Journal of Epidemiology* 119(1), 33–43, 1984. (NIOSH-00140953)

37. Pratt, P.C. "Chronic respiratory impairment in long-term cotton workers: Relationship to smoking: Reversibility," *Proceedings of the Eighth Cotton Dust Research Conference,* Beltwide Cotton Production Research Conferences, pp. 26–28, 1984. (NIOSH-00147917)

38. Saccomanno, G., C. Yale, W. Dixon, O. Auerbach, and G.C. Huth. "An epidemiological analysis of the relationship between exposure to Rn progeny, smoking and bronchogenic carcinoma in the U-mining population of the Colorado Plateau—1960–1980," *Health Physics* 50(5), 605–618, 1986. (NIOSH-00159283)

39. Damber, L., and L.-G. Larsson. "Underground mining, smoking, and lung cancer: A case-control study in the iron ore municipalities in Northern Sweden," *Journal of the National Cancer Institute* 74(6), 1207–1213, 1985. (NIOSH-00149783)

40. Edling, C. "Radon daughter exposure in mines, smoking and lung cancer," *Archiv za Higijenu Rada i Toksikologiju* 34(4), 265–273, 1983. (NIOSH-00147699)

41. Lundin, F.E., Jr., J.W. Lloyd, E.M. Smith, V.E. Archer, and D.A. Holaday. "Mortality of uranium miners in relation to radiation exposure, hard-rock mining and cigarette smoking—1950 through September 1967," *Health Physics* 16, 571–578, 1969. (NIOSH-00128792)

3

Employer Considerations and Workplace Smoking

Workplace smoking, or any smoking, for that matter, has an impact on the health of the worker. The impact may not be felt for many years, and some never seem to suffer any ill effects. For others, the effects of smoking, and of ETS for the involuntary smoker, are immediate: the smoker may feel ill, may cough, or have trouble recovering from seemingly trivial respiratory illnesses. The involuntary smoker may cough or have dry throat from inhaling the smoke, or may have an asthma attack, if so disposed. These effects are not unexpected for respiratory mucosa exposed to particulates and chemicals.

Smoking has other subtle effects. The lungs are directly affected by smoking; it is well known that champion athletes are expected to abstain from smoking, lest their wind be cut. Long-distance swimmers who smoke have trouble with shortened breath, which could be a danger to them, as it could also be to those who dive without breathing equipment. The workplace can also be a hazard to the smoker and the involuntary smoker, and, in turn, the smoking worker can also endanger the workplace.

Smoking costs money. Smoking causes lost time due to ill health; compromises the health and comfort of workers; causes work incapacity; interferes with exercise routines; causes accidents; compromises fitness; and limits the ability of the worker to perform certain tasks. Each of these problems will be examined in turn.

COSTS OF SMOKING

It has been estimated that the economic consequences of cigarette smoking in the United States reached $27.5 billion in 1976; of this amount, lost production was $19.1 billion, direct health care costs were $8.2 billion, and fire losses were $0.2 billion. The per capita cost of illness related to smoking was calculated to be $459. Using 1980 dollars, the annual cost of cigarette smoking has been estimated to be $47.5 billion; $11 billion is attributed to excess medical expenses incurred by smokers and $36.5 billion to early death, premature retirement, and losses due to absenteeism. Costs of illness to nonsmokers exposed to smoke was not considered.

Annual costs of smoking to the average employer have been estimated as ranging from $336 to $624 in 1980 dollars per average smoking employee. These costs have been further broken down into $274 for excess insurance costs, $80 for absenteeism, $166 for reduced productivity, and $104 for involuntary smoker impact. Smokers average 33% to 45% more absenteeism than do nonsmokers; the 1979 Surgeon General's report indicated that smoking employees use 50% more sick leave.

Total costs of allowing smoking at the workplace have been estimated by other researchers to be as high as $4,611 per smoker per year. Regardless of what figures are used, it is clear that allowing smoking at the workplace is expensive to employers. The business reasons for adopting restrictive smoking policies are compelling since health care expenses, which are borne substantially by the employer, have risen dramatically over the last few years. Also, labor and production costs have increased, futher exacerbating the excess absenteeism, on-the-job down time, and maintenance burdens associated with workplace smoking. The employed smoker also imposes a much greater maintenance burden on the employer for cleaning, repairing, repainting, and replacing furnishings and equipment. Clearly, there are savings of all kinds for an employer when employees do not smoke.

SMOKING PREVALENCE IN THE WORKPLACE: EMPLOYEE CHARACTERISTICS

Before characterizing the smoking behavior of the U.S. adult workforce, it will be useful to describe the patterns of employment for men and women. Men are more likely to be employed in professional, technical, management, and blue-collar occupations (although this mix is changing); women are more likely to be employed in professional, technical, clerical, and service occupations, or to be homemakers. Although there was an increase in participation by women in white-collar occupations between 1970 and 1980, the ranking of occupational categories by their relative frequency for both sexes remained about the same in 1980 as it did in 1970. Because of their low relative frequency, farm, sales, and clerical workers, laborers, and service workers have less impact on the smoking behavior of the total male workforce, and female farm workers, laborers, craftsmen and kindred workers, sales workers, managers, and administrators have a modest impact on the smoking behavior of the total female workforce.

Smoking Prevalence

Surveys have repeatedly shown that blue-collar workers are more likely than white-collar workers to smoke cigarettes. Recent estimates from National Health Interview Surveys (NHIS) continue to substantiate this finding. Overall, smoking rates for blue-collar men (47.1%) exceed that of white-collar men (33.0%). The same pattern holds for women, but is less pronounced, with smoking rates among blue-collar women (38.1%) exceeding that of white-collar women (31.9%). Among women, this white-collar—blue-collar difference exists only for the younger age group (aged 20 to 44); for older women (aged 45 to 64) there is virtually no difference in smoking prevalence between these two categories of workers.

For men, the highest rates of current smoking occur among craftsmen and kindred workers, operatives and kindred workers, laborers, service workers, and the unemployed. The lowest smoking rates for men occur among professional, technical, and kindred workers, managers and administrators, clerical and kindred workers, and farm workers.

For women 20 to 64 years of age, the highest smoking rates are found among craftsmen and kindred workers, and managers and adminstrators. Among women 20 to 44 years of age, there are also relatively high smoking rates among operatives and kindred workers, service workers, and the unemployed. The lowest rates of current smoking occur among professional, technical, and kindred workers, regardless of age. For homemakers, the category representing nearly 42% of all women aged 20 to 64, the prevalence of smoking among those aged 20 to 44 is midway between the prevalence rates for white-collar and blue-collar occupations. However, among women 45 to 64 years of age, smoking rates vary little by occupational group (with the single exception of managers and administrators), with white-collar workers, blue-collar workers, and homemakers all having approximately the same smoking prevalence.

Among men, a more detailed breakdown of smoking by occupation shows that painters, truck drivers, construction workers, carpenters, auto mechanics, and guards and watchmen have the highest rates of current smoking (among occupations having 100 or more cases in the 1978–1980 NHIS), each exceeding 50%. In contrast, electrical and electronic engineers, lawyers, and secondary school teachers have the lowest rates of current smoking, all under 25%. (No mention is made of smoking behavior in occupations such as waiters, nursing personnel, elementary school teachers, food service workers, bank tellers, or tailoring workers, occupations generally thought to be traditionally female areas.)

Among women, waitresses have a noticeably higher rate of current smoking than other groups, followed by cashiers, assemblers, nurses' aides, machine operators, practical nurses, and packers and wrappers—all of whom have rates of current smoking that equal or surpass 40%. The lowest rates of smoking occur among women employed as elementary school teachers, food service workers, bank tellers, and sewing-oriented workers. (No mention is made of women employed in the electrical and electronic industries, or as lawyers, secondary school teachers, and other traditional male occupations mentioned above.)

Because of the exemplar role of doctors and nurses in regard to health, their smoking rates are of special interest. Although the sample is relatively small, doctors have among the lowest rates of current smoking (18.1%). Among nurses, the pattern of smoking reflects the white-collar—service worker distinction; registered nurses have among the lowest rates of current smoking, but practical nurses have among the highest rates. (No information is available on the smoking practices of male nurses; the information presented here is presumed to be about female nurses. The smoking behavior of doctors available from sources quoted here is presumed to include female doctors.)

ette Consumption

cupational differences in cigarette consumption the same patterns observed for prevalence. On the average, adult male white-collar smokers consume 24 cigarettes per day, essentially the same as the number of cigarettes consumed by blue-collar smokers. In virtually all occupational subgroups, adult men report an average daily consumption exceeding 20 cigarettes. Consumption levels are highest among managers, administrators, and sales workers. These numbers represent daily cigarette consumption and need to be interpreted with some caution, as there may be a substantial underreporting of cigarette consumption, and the tendency to underreport may not be constant across occupational categories.

For women, no difference in consumption is found between white-collar and blue-collar smokers. On the average, white-collar female smokers consume 19.5 cigarettes per day, compared with 19.8 cigarettes per day for blue-collar smokers, 19.4 cigarettes for homemakers, and 19.0 cigarettes for service workers. Female smokers employed as managers or administrators, or craftsmen and kindred workers, report the highest consumption levels, averaging more than 20 cigarettes per day; women employed in professional, technical, or kindred occupations report lower average daily consumption. However, as in the case of the men, these differences are not large, averaging fewer than 2 to 4 cigarettes per day.

The higher the average daily consumption of cigarettes within an occupational group, the more likely it is that this group will also contain a higher percentage of heavy smokers (more than 20 or more than 40 cigarettes a day). Overall, 72% of the male smokers employed in white-collar occupations reported smoking more than 20 cigarettes a day, and over 21% reported smoking 40 or more cigarettes a day. Comparable figures for blue-collar smokers are 72% and 18%, respectively.

Among adult women, the percentage of heavy smokers is generally lower than for men, with women employed as craftsmen or kindred workers reporting higher percentages of heavy smoking than other female occupational groups. The pattern for homemakers closely parallels that of white-collar workers, but service workers have slightly lower rates of heavy smoking than white-collar workers. For both men and women, and across virtually all occupational groups, smokers 45 years of age or older are more likely to report a higher percentage of heavy smokers than their 20- to 44-year old counterparts.

Age of Initiation of Smoking

Men employed as blue-collar workers initiate smoking approximately 14 months earlier, on the average, than men employed in white-collar occupations. The earliest ages of initiation are reported by men employed as laborers (16.5 years), operatives or kindred workers (16.6 years), or craftsmen and kindred workers (16.8 years). Men employed in professional, technical, or kindred occupations, or as managers or administrators, sales workers, or clerical or kindred workers report later onset of smoking, ranging between 17.7 and 18.1 years of age.

For women, blue-collar and service workers report a somewhat earlier onset of smoking than white-collar workers or homemakers (about 6 months earlier). The earliest age of initiation occurs among women employed as laborers (17.4 years), and the latest age of initiation occurs among women employed in professional, technical, or kindred occupations (19.4 years). Across all occupational categories, men report an earlier age of initiation than women; this difference is most pronounced within the 45 to 64 age group.

An important inference of the age of initiation reported by workers is that a substantial fraction of smokers report beginning to smoke at ages when they would be first entering the workforce. This suggests that a set of influences that promote initiation may be present in the initial socialization into the workforce.

Because cigarette smoking usually begins between the ages of 12 and 25, the prevalence of smoking among people 25 years of age or older is determined in large part by the rate at which they stop smoking (or die). The percentage of former smokers (as a portion of "ever smoked") by occupational group uncovered a few surprises. For men, relatively higher percentages of former smokers are found among professional, technical, and kindred workers (55.2%) and managers and administrators (47.7%)—the same occupational groups reporting lower rates of current smoking. The striking feature for women is the uniformly lower percentage of former smokers when compared with men. However, even here the same general pattern can be found; occupations that have lower rates of current smoking also tend to have a higher percentage of former smokers. In general, there are substantial differences by occupational category, with white-collar workers of both sexes having a higher percentage of former smokers than have blue-collar workers. This white-collar—blue-collar difference is most pronounced among men. Among women, homemakers tend to mirror the pattern of white-collar women.

It does not appear that the lower percentage of former smokers in blue-collar occupations occurs simply because blue-collar workers are less likely than white-collar workers to attempt to quit. Among men, white-collar current smokers are more likely to report "a serious attempt" to quit smoking, but these differences are typically only half as large as the white-collar—blue-collar differences in the proportion of former smokers. Among women, the white-collar—blue-collar differences are relatively small and show a mixed pattern.

Recent Changes in Smoking Behavior

A comparison of smoking estimates for the period 1970–1980 reveals several interesting changes by occupational group and sex. Among men, there was a 19% proportional decline in smoking prevalence between 1970 and 1980 for white-collar workers (40.8% vs. 33.0%), compared with a 14% decline for blue-collar workers (55.0 vs. 47.1%). Occupations with the largest decline in male smoking include professional, technical, and kindred occupations (21% decline) and farm workers (20.7%); the unemployed (3.6%) and service workers (10.9%)

had the smallest proportionate declines in smoking prevalence.

Among white-collar women, there was a proportionate reduction in smoking prevalence of 11.6% between 1970 and 1980 (36.1% vs. 31.9%), but blue-collar women showed virtually no change in smoking prevalence (1.0% proportionate increase).

The greater rate of decline in smoking prevalence for men has produced two fundamental changes in the occupational smoking patterns in this country. In 1970, men employed in professional, technical, or kindred occupations, or as managers or administrators, had a higher rate of smoking than their female counterparts. By the end of the decade, this pattern had been reversed; a slightly higher percentage of women in these two occupational groups now smoke cigarettes. If the previous 10-year trends prevail, by the end of this decade women are likely to reach parity with men in the prevalence of smoking among blue-collar workers (as an aggregate) and clerical and kindred workers, and to surpass men in smoking prevalence in two additional occupational categories: craftsmen and kindred workers, and laborers.

Only one specific occupational group for men showed a net gain in smoking prevalence between 1970 and 1980 (electricians), but painters, farm laborers, stock clerks and storekeepers, and deliverymen and routemen had net reductions in excess of 10 percentage points. Among women, three occupational groups showed a net increase in smoking prevalence between 1970 and 1980 (practical nurses, cashiers, and packers and wrappers), but relatively large net declines in smoking prevalence occurred among receptionists, waitresses, bank tellers, secretaries, and hairdressers and cosmetologists.

The 10-year changes in daily consumption patterns show that among white-collar men, there was a 1.8% proportionate increase in the percentage of smokers who averaged 20 or more cigarettes per day, compared with a 3.3% increase for blue-collar men. Professional, technical, and kindred workers, clerical and kindred workers, and the unemployed showed a net decrease in the percentage of smokers of 20 or more cigarettes per day. The overall pattern is one of modest differences.

For women, the proportionate increase in number of smokers of 20 or more cigarettes per day was 7.4% for white-collar workers (55.3% vs. 59.4%) and 4.8% for homemakers (56.4% vs. 59.1%). Service workers showed virtually no change between 1970 and 1980. Among blue-collar women, however, the proportionate increase in smokers of 20 or more cigarettes per day was a much larger 20.4% (51.5% vs. 62.0%). High proportionate increases in 20-plus smokers occurred among women employed as operatives or kindred workers (37.8%) or craftsmen or kindred workers (33.2%). If these 10-year trends continue, by the end of this decade female blue-collar smokers may surpass their male counterparts in the percentage classified as moderate to heavy smokers (smoking more than 20 cigarettes daily).

Among men, the net change in smokers averaging more than 40 cigarettes a day generally parallels that of 20-plus smokers. Only the unemployed show a net decrease in the percentage of current smokers averaging 40 or more cigarettes per day. Among women, the net changes in heavy smoking between 1970 and 1980 are relatively modest.

Race

Among black men, there are almost twice as many blue-collar workers as there are white-collar workers. This is in contrast with white men, who fall about equally into the white-collar and blue-collar categories. Additionally, blacks of both sexes are more heavily concentrated in the service category of workers, making this category an important one to consider when examining occupational differences in smoking by race. Black men are also twice as likely as white men to fall into the unemployed category, which includes both unemployed people and those "not in the labor force."

The differences in smoking prevalence between black men and white men parallel the differences between blue-collar and white-collar workers, with black men having a considerably higher smoking prevalence (47.7%) than white men (40.2%). Among men, blue-collar workers have considerably higher smoking rates than white-collar workers within each racial group, with black male blue-collar workers having the highest smoking prevalence (52.1%).

Among black women, there is little difference in smoking prevalence between occupations, although homemakers have a somewhat higher smoking rate. However, among white women, the expected white-collar—blue-collar, service worker differences prevail, with blue-collar and service workers having a higher smoking prevalence (39.6% and 38.7%, respectively) than white-collar workers (32.0%).

Black workers are considerably less likely than their white counterparts to be heavy smokers (smoking 20 or more cigarettes daily). This holds true for all categories of workers and for men and women. Among white women and black men, blue-collar workers are somewhat more likely than others to be heavy smokers. The consumption differences between white workers and black workers are even more pronounced when the percentage of smokers smoking 40 or more cigarettes daily is examined. White men are about 4 times more likely than black men to smoke 40 or more cigarettes daily, regardless of occupation. Similarly, white women are about 3 times more likely than black women to smoke more than 40 cigarettes daily, regardless of occupational group.

Among women, there are minimal racial or occupational differences in the proportion of current smokers who have attempted to quit smoking. However, blue-collar, service, and unemployed black men are somewhat less likely than all other groups to have attempted to quit. Among those who have ever smoked, white-collar male workers are the most likely to have quit smoking. Blue-collar and service workers generally have lower quit rates than white-collar workers, and this pattern holds true for white men, black men, and white women. Black women have low quit rates regardless of occupational category. Additionally, black male blue-collar workers have a considerably lower quit rate (24.9%) than white male blue-collar workers (36.0%).

In summary, black workers are more likely than white workers to be cigarette smokers, with black male blue-collar workers having the highest smoking rate. In contrast, white workers are much more likely than black workers to be heavy smokers, regardless of job category. White workers are more likely to have quit smoking, with the exception of white female blue-collar workers. Black male blue-collar workers and all black female workers have low quit rates. Among black men, white men, and white women, white-collar workers have both lower rates of current smoking and higher proportions of former smokers than do blue-collar or service workers. The one group that deviates from this pattern is black women; white-collar workers have a higher rate of current smoking and a somewhat lower proportion of former smokers than do blue-collar or service workers, and homemakers have a relatively high rate of current smoking.

ECONOMICS OF HEALTH PROBLEMS RELATED TO SMOKING

Smokers take more sick time than nonsmokers, according to a study reported in 1986.[1] Stresses cause smokers to smoke more; in a study made on nursing students who smoked, the students who reported that they were likely to smoke in a stressful situation adapted less well to the stress of hospital duties.[2] A British study found that changes in the demand for medical services could be related to tobacco consumption levels.[3] This last study also surveyed the health problems suffered by smokers who no longer smoke, but have long-term health problems from the earlier smoking habit. Finally, a study made in 1984 determined that, simply, smokers were more often disabled than nonsmokers, especially in age groups under 40 years of age.[4]

HEALTH AND COMFORT OF WORKERS

Nonsmoking employees report annoyance and irritation as effects of ETS exposure; frustration and hostility may also be the result of smoke exposure. Employees subjected to ETS may characterize their workplace air as "bad" with regard to ETS, and eye irritation as well as irritation of respiratory tract and throat mucosa have been reported.[5] Smokers have experienced changes in numbers, types, and functions of respiratory epithelial and inflammatory cells, setting the stage for later emphysema, chronic brochitis, and cancers of the respiratory tract; there is evidence that these diseases may also affect nonsmokers in the same manner, via the inhalation of ETS. It is distinctly possible that all the disorders afflicting smokers also affect nonsmokers, due to the inhalation of tobacco smoke. Smoking has been associated with an increased risk of hearing loss in noise exposed individuals.[6] Studies on the interactions between prescription drugs and smoking showed that several of these interactions were responsible for higher accident rates, increased absenteeism, and lost productivity. And, finally, the effect of smokers on nonsmokers showed increasing incidences of clashes that affected work harmony and productivity.[7]

Work Capacity

Smoking affects various nervous system responses; time estimation performance changes in visual processing tasks.[8] Peripheral vision field is larger in nonsmokers than in smokers under conditions of low illumination.[9,10] There are two lengthy bibliographies in the literature on the effects of cigarette smoking and nicotine on human performance.[11,12] Field-dependence and contrast sensitivity were measured in smokers and nonsmokers; the nonsmokers were better able to judge contrasts, particularly important in aircraft and vehicle operators.[13] The effects of smoking withdrawal on complex formance and physiological responses were ated aircraft cabin altitude of 6,500 feet, with es and decline of tracking capabilities deter- sults of smoking deprivation.[14,15]

Exercise, Fitness, and Smoking

The immediate effect of smoking of moderate intensity is impairment of the cardiovascular system; significantly higher carboxyhemoglobin concentrations were found in smokers after a resting pulmonary function test was made.[16] Carboxyhemoglobin is the union of carbon monoxide with hemoglobin; the carbon monoxide molecule is more likely to replace oxygen on hemoglobin, because the chemical bond between hemoglobin and carbon monoxide is stronger than that between oxygen and hemoglobin, and as a result carbon monoxide will be preferentially carried to the lungs. The hemoglobin will not release the carbon monoxide molecule until it returns to the lungs, therefore depriving the body, especially the brain, of needed oxygen.

A Navy study found that smoking had a clear negative impact on physical fitness, most notably on cardiorespiratory endurance and muscular endurance. Navy personnel who had never smoked were leaner, could do more sit-ups, and scored higher on the overall physical fitness rating than current and former smokers.[17] Another Navy study found that divers who have relatively heavy smoking histories may be at greater risk for developing significant decline in pulmonary function, and diving exposure factors other than years of diving could contribute to the risk.[18] Smoking increases the heart rate.[19]

Accidents and Smoking

A Spanish study performed in 1973 found that a positive relationship exists between smoking and accidents; the researchers theorized that psychic distraction is related to a desynchronizing effect on the central nervous system and the attentional needs of the smoking act, creating the situations that lead to accidents.[20] The workers in this study were operating machinery in a factory.

DEPOSITION AND ABSORPTION OF TOBACCO SMOKE CONSTITUENTS

An understanding of the deposition of cigarette smoke particles in the respiratory tract is important because many of the toxic constituents of cigarette smoker are contained in the particles. The quantity retained, which constitutes the dose, is some fraction of the quantity inhaled. Measures of tobacco smoke constituents or their metabolites are also important because they reflect the absorption of tobacco smoke by the individual smoker or nonsmoker, and therefore may be more accurate markers of actual exposure experienced by an individual. There is little experimental information describing the deposition of ETS in the respiratory tract; however, cigarette smoke particles probably behave similarly to other inhaled particles. In contrast, there are a number of observations of different markers in the biological fluids of smokers and nonsmokers. This short review discusses particle deposition and factors affecting deposition, biologic markers of smoke absorption, and levels of the markers found in smokers and nonsmokers.

Deposition

In this review, the term "deposition" refers to the transfer of a particle from inhaled air to the surface of any portion of the respiratory tract, from nose to alveolus. "Retention" is the quantity of deposited material remaining in the respiratory tract at a specified time following deposition. Retention decreases as clearance mechanisms reduce the respiratory tract burden of inhaled particles.

An aerosol is a suspension of particles in a gaseous or vapor medium; cigarette smoke is an aerosol. The smaller particles of an aerosol, despite their relatively small mass, have a large total surface area because of their great number. Both total deposition and deposition site in the respiratory tract vary substantially with particle size.

Size Distribution

One of the reasons for discussing size distribution and respiratory tract deposition of particles is to illustrate the discrepancy between measured particle size of mainstream smoke and its measured deposition in the human respiratory tract. The deposition fraction is several times higher than would be predicted on the basis of its particulate size. Measured deposition of sidestream smoke is more in keeping with its measured particle size.

Size distribution of diluted mainstream smoke aerosol from a laboratory smoke generator (designed to operate similarly to a human smoker) is measured by a variety of techniques such as light scattering, microscopic examination, or impactor collection device. Experiments have revealed that there is an ultrafine component (below 0.1 micrometer in size) to cigarette smoke. These very fine particles have been shown to have a different chemistry than those of the larger particles.

Laboratory methods used to study mainstream smoke are highly artificial and may not accurately duplicate the generation, dilution, and inhalation of this type of smoke; smoking technique and respiratory tract conditions may promote changes in particle size. Smoking techniques differ between smokers, and may be changed due to health considerations or how long the puff is held before exhalation. These techniques can change the amount of particle coagulation that occurs within the respiratory tract, and therefore reduce the number of very small particles that are ultimately exhaled. Also, the accumulation of water in or on the particles in the high humidity of the respiratory tract can increase particle diameter, possibly as much as 30%. Coagulation and water uptake by particles in the respiratory tract may considerably alter particle size distributions so that measurements under laboratory conditions probably do not represent distributions found in actual mainstream smoking conditions.

Sidestream smoke is generated by cigarettes burning spontaneously between puffs and is quantitatively the major contributor to ETS. Fifty-five percent of the tobacco in a cigarette is burned between puffs to form sidestream smoke. Dilution takes place as smoke rises in ambient air currents. This dilution reduces, but probably does not eliminate entirely, the coagulation that causes the particles to increase in size, as they might in mainstream smoke. The size distribution of sidestream smoke might be expected to resemble that of diluted mainstream smoke.

Particle Deposition in the Respiratory Tract

Total deposition has been studied both theoretically and experimentally. The major property to be considered is particle size and its influence on impaction, sedimentation, and diffusion. Inertial impaction is the mechanism that causes particles moving in an airstream to be unable, because of excessive mass, to follow the airstream around a bend. Large particles impact at the bend in the airstream or in the lung or near a site of airway branching. The larger the particle, the greater is its chance of depositing by impaction. The effect of gravity on suspended particles causes them to fall, a process called sedimentation. Sedimentation and impaction are relatively unimportant processes for particles smaller than 0.5 micrometer. Diffusion is the net transport of particles caused by Brownian motion, and becomes increasingly important for particles less than 0.5 micrometer in size. The mass median diameter of sidestream smoke is in the 0.3–0.5 micrometer size range; total deposition for inhaled particles is in the 10% to 30% range for 0.5 micrometer sized particles.

Respiratory patterns clearly affect particle deposition; most important for all particles, including ETS, is the residence time in the lung. Deposition increases with slow deep inspiration and with breath holding. This indicates that deposition of ETS during involuntary smoking increases with the increasing activity level of the exposed individual, which also involves increased oxygen consumption.

The presence of an electrical charge on particles may increase deposition; mainstream smoke is highly charged. The addition of either a positive or negative charge to inhaled particles increases deposition (from animal studies), and neutralization of the charge reduces deposition by about 21%. Particle growth by water absorption may also affect deposition. Mathematical models have predicted a considerable size change for some particles during transit in the humid respiratory tract, changes that could significantly alter deposition.

Many reports have described the measured deposition of mainstream cigarette smoke in the human respiratory tract. Although few studies of total sidestream smoke deposition are available, those few suggest that sidestream smoke does indeed deposit in a manner similar to that found for laboratory-designed research aerosols. Deposition for sidestream smoke has been measured in mouth-breathing human volunteers to be 11%. ETS exposure frequently occurs with breathing through the nose rather than through the mouth, and the fraction of 0.2 micrometer size particles deposited is similar for both mouth and nose breathing.

Total deposition is subdivided into the fractions depositing in the upper respiratory tract (larynx and above), the tracheobronchial region (trachea to and including terminal bronchioles), and the pulmonary region (respiratory bronchioles and beyond). Deposition in these areas is referred to as regional deposition; particle size is a major determinant of both total and regional deposition.

The regional deposition of mainstream cigarette smoke in smokers, studied using tracer methods, has been shown to be less than 40% in the pulmonary region, compared with an expected 90% for 0.5 micrometer particles (size for cigarette smoke). This finding supports the concept that mainstream smoke particles increase in size in the respiratory tract by coagulation or other mechanisms, and that this growth affects total and regional deposition. Deposition is probably not uniform within a lung region; the mass deposited in the airways, for instance, may vary widely. Enhanced deposition at certain anatomic sites may be important for some inhaled species; for instance, the concentration of carcinogens at a site may favor the site for cancer development. This may be especially important for cigarette smoke, because lung cancer may occur at sites of high deposition such as airway bifurcations.

Epidemiological studies of the pathophysiologic consequences of involuntary smoking have emphasized, among other things, an increase in the incidence of respiratory illness in children. Tracheobronchial depositions per kilogram body weight for 5 micrometer particles has been estimated to be 6 times higher in the resting newborn infant than in a resting adult. Tracheobronchial deposition in infancy for sidestream smoke particles has been predicted to be 2 to 3 times higher than for adults. Total deposition is also predicted to be higher for infants than for adults.

Respiratory Tract Dose of Environmental Tobacco Smoke

The dose of ETS to the respiratory tract is the product of the amount of smoke inhaled and the deposition fraction; to estimate dose, the content of smoke in inhaled air must be known as well as respiratory minute volume, defined as the volume of breath inhaled or exhaled per minute. Sidestream smoke concentrations have been measured at 2 to 4 mg/m^3 for rooms of 140 m^3 in size containing from 50 to 70 persons. Such levels exceed the EPA air quality standards for total suspended particulates of 75 micrograms/m^3 annual average and the 260 microgram/m^3 24-hour average in the United States and the 250 microgram/m^3 24-hour average for thc United Kingdom.

Measurements of ETS concentrations vary widely depending on location and measurement techniques. Levels of total suspended particulates (TSP) measured under realistic circumstances have ranged from 20 to 60 micrograms/m^3 in no-smoking areas, and can range from 100 to 700 micrograms/m^3 in the presence of smokers. These measurements include all suspended particulates, and so could include particles other than tobacco smoke. However, in a smoking indoor setting where measurements as high as 600 micrograms/m^3 were found, tobacco smoke is the major contributor to particle mass, with the non-tobacco smoke contribution being small and similar to that measured in a no-smoking area. ETS levels have been estimated to be from 20 to 480 micrograms/m^3 in bus and airline waiting rooms, and as high as 640 micrograms/m^3 in cocktail lounges. These calculations are based on an average weighted nicotine fraction of 2.6%, an approach that may underestimate tobacco smoke particulate concentration.

Mass deposition in the respiratory tract can be estimated if the atmospheric burden of cigarette smoke particulates, minute volume, and deposition fraction is known. Assuming a smoke concentration of 500 micrograms/m^3, a volume of 12 liters per minute, and a deposition fraction of 11%, mass deposition over an 8-hour work shift would be 0.317 mg.

Evaluation of Smoking-Related Cancers in the Workplace

Cigarette smoking and occupational exposures may interact biologically, within a given statistical model and in their public health consequences. The demonstration of an interaction at one of these levels does not always characterize the nature of the interaction at the other levels. Information on smoking behavior should be collected as part of the health screening of all workers and made a part of their permanent exposure record. Examination of the smoking behavior of an exposed population should include measures of smoking prevalence, smoking dose, and duration of smoking. Differences in age of onset of exposure to cigarette smoke and occupational exposures should be considered when evaluating studies of occupational exposure, particularly when the exposed population is relatively young or the exposure is of relatively recent onset.

Evaluation of Chronic Lung Disease in the Workplace

Existing resources for monitoring the occurrence of occupational lung diseases are not comprehensive and do not include information on cigarette smoking. Other approaches, such as registries, might offer more accurate data and facilitate research related to occupational lung diseases. In studies on occupational lung diseases, emphasis should be placed on measures of physiological change, X-ray detectable abnormality, and other objective measures, Because of the variability in diagnostic criteria for chronic lung disease. Further studies that correlate lung function with histopathology should be carried out in occupationally exposed smokers and non-smokers. The effects of chest x-rays should be clarified. In particular, the sensitivity of the ILO classification to smoking-related changes should be further evaluated in healthy populations.

To determine if smoking is reported with bias by occupationally exposed workers, self-reported histories should be compared with biological markers of smoking in appropriate populations. Mechanisms through which specific occupational agents and cigarette smoking might interact should be systematically considered. Both laboratory and epidemiological approaches should be used to evaluate such interactions. Statistical methods for evaluating interactions require further development. In particular, the biological implications of conventional modeling approaches should be explored. Further, the limitations posed by sample size for examining independent and interactive effects should be evaluated. The consequences of misclassification by exposure estimates and of the colinearity of exposure variables should also be addressed.

The role of cigarette smoking in the "healthy worker effect" requires further evaluation. Approaches for apportioning the impairment in a specific individual between occupational causes and cigarette smoking should be developed and validated.

REFERENCES

1. Van Tuinen, M., and G. Land. "Smoking and excess sick leave in a department of health," *Journal of Occupational Medicine* 28(1), 33–35, 1986. (NIOSH-00157740)

2. Parkes, K.R. "Smoking as a moderator of the relationship between affective state and absence from work," *Journal of Applied Psychology* 68(4), 698–708, 1983. (NIOSH-00138526)

3. Atkinson, A.B., and T.W. Meade. "Methods and preliminary findings in assessing the economic and health services consequences of smoking, with particular reference to lung cancer," *Journal of the Royal Statistical Society* 136, 297–312, 1974. (NTIS HRP-0011060/1)

4. Kozak, J.T. "Contribution of smoking habit to work incapacity," *Bulletin of the Industrial Union Against Tuberculosis* 59(1–2), 48–49, 1984. (NIOSH-00153741)

5. *Health Consequences of Involuntary Smoking: A Report of the Surgeon General.* U.S. Department of Health and Human Services, Public Health Service. Washington, DC: Superintendent of Documents, U.S. Government Printing Office, 1986. 359 pp. DHHS(CDC)87-8398. pp. 7, 231, 239.

6. Barone, J.A., J.M. Peters, D.H. Garabrant, L. Bernstein, and R. Krebsbach. "Smoking as a risk factor in noise-reduced hearing loss," *Journal of Occupational Medicine* 29(9), 741–745, 1987. (NIOSH-)0174055)

7. Blackwood, M.J. "Health risks of smoking increased by exposure to workplace chemicals," *Occupational Health and Safety* 54(2), 23–24, 26–27, 81, 1985. (NIOSH-00145316)

8. Breidenbach, Steven T., James L. Arnold, and Norman W. Heimstra. *The Effects of Smoking on Time Estimation Performance.* Vermillion, SD: University of South Dakota, 1976. 69 pp. (NTIS AD-A047744/8)

9. Heimstra, Norman W. *The Effects of Smoking on Peripheral Movement Detection and Time Estimation Performance.* Vermillion, SD: Univeristy of South Dakota, 1977. 9 pp. (NTIS AD-A052693/9)

10. Scoughton, Craig R., and Norman W. Heimstra. *The Effects of Smoking on Peripheral Movement Detection.* Vermillion, SD: University of South Dakota, 1973. 50 pp. (NTIS AD-778 928/2)

11. Millis, R.M. *Review of the Scientific Literature and Preparation of an Annotated Bibliography on Effects of Cigarette Smoking and Nicotine on Human Performance*. Volume 1. Washington, DC: Associate Consultants, Inc., 1986. 187 pp. (NTIS AD-A186805/8/XAB)

12. Millis, R.M. *Review of the Scientific Literature and Preparation of an Annotated Bibliography on Effects of Cigarette Smoking and Nicotine on Human Performance*. Volume 2. Washington, DC: Associate Consultants, Inc., 1985. 156 pp. (NTIS AD-A186806/6/XAB)

13. Fine, Bernard J., and John L. Kobrick. *Cigarette Smoking, Field-Dependence and Contrast Sensitivity*. Natick, MA: Army Research Inst. of Environmental Medicine, 1986. 24 pp. (NTIS AD-A173450/8/XAB)

14. Mertens, Henry W., Jess M. McKenzie, and E. Arnold Higgins. *Some Effects of Smoking Withdrawal on Complex Performance and Physiological Responses*. Washington, DC: Federal Aviation Administration, 1983. 18 pp. (NTIS AD-A126551/1)

15. Gibson, Richard S., and William F. Moroney. *A Limited Review of the Effect of Cigarette Smoking on Performance with Emphasis on Aviation*. Pensacola, FL: Naval Aerospace Medical Inst., 1972. 12 pp. (NTIS AD-754 421)

16. Hirsch, G.L., D.Y. Sue, K. Wasserman, T.E. Robinson, and J.E. Hansen. "Immediate effects of cigarette smoking on cardiorespiratory responses to exercise," *Journal of Applied Physiology* 58(6), 1975–1981, 1985. (NIOSH-00149470)

17. Conway, T.L., T.A. Cronan. *Smoking and Physical Fitness Among Navy Shipboard Personnel*. San Diego, CA: Naval Health Research Center, 1986. 21 pp. (NTIS AD-A180160/4/XAB)

18. Dembert, M.L., G.J. Beck, J.F. Jekel, and L.W. Mooney. "Relations of smoking and diving experience to pulmonary function among U.S. Navy divers," *Undersea Biomedical Research*, 11(3), 299–304, 1984. (NTIS AD-A164481/4/XAB)

19. Burse, Richard L., Ralph F. Goldman, Elliot Danforth, Jr., Edward S. Horton, and Ethan A.H. Sims. *Effects of Cigarette Smoking on Body Weight, Energy Expenditure, Appetite and Endocrine Function*. Natick, MA: Army Research Inst. of Environmental Medicine, 1982. 29 pp. (NTIS AD-A114213/2)

20. Yuste, P.C., and M.L. de Guevara. "The influence of smoking on work accidents. Statistical survey," *Medicina y Seguridad del Trabajo* 21(84), 38–46, 1973. (NIOSH-00104258)

4

Workplace Restrictions on Smoking: Decisions and Policymaking

Since the 1970s, evidence on health risks of involuntary smoking has been accompanied by social action regulating smoking in public places. The action has been designed to protect individuals from exposure to sidestream smoke by regulating the circumstances in which smoking is permitted. Government action has been the technique used; at state and local levels, legislation has been employed; agency rulings predominate at the federal level. Relatively little judicial action restricts smoking in public; most cases have dealt with nonsmokers' rights to smoke-free workplaces. The private sector has gained advantages since the 1970s; businesses have adopted smoking policies to protect worker health, restaurants have adopted nonsmoking areas, hospitals restrict smoking, and hotels and motels offer nonsmoking rooms.

Although this trend is the result of growing evidence about the health effects smoking, both involuntary and voluntary, it also reflects changing public attitudes about smoking. In 1964, the Surgeon General's report on cigarette smoking called attention to health hazards, and since that time the acceptability of public smoking has declined. A majority of the public now supports the right of nonsmokers to breathe clean, smoke-free air and favors legislation or policies to enforce that right.

CURRENT POLICIES DEALING WITH SMOKING IN PUBLIC

A public place is defined as any enclosed area in which the public is permitted or to which the public is invited. Smoking restrictions are generally limited to indoor enclosed spaces. Since this definition is necessarily broad, a diverse group of facilities are included which differ in the degree to which smoking is restricted, the ease with which new rules can be introduced, and in the methods with which new rulings can be proposed and adopted. The extent and acceptability of smoking restrictions in public areas is influenced by whether ownership is public or private; whether or not smoking was previously permitted; the degree to which persons are exposed to involuntary smoking (determined by facility size, ventilation, and separation of smokers from nonsmokers); and the degree of inconvenience that smoking restrictions pose to smokers. Smoking restrictions are least controversial in facilities where traditional prohibition of smoking has been the rule, such as in theaters or libraries, or where smoking would be inappropriate, such as health care facilities or gyms. Small areas such as elevators or transit vehicles usually are subject to smoking restrictions. However, a strong association exists between eating and drinking and smoking; smoking restrictions have been difficult to obtain in restaurants and bars.

STATE LAWS REGULATING SMOKING

Most legislation restricting smoking has been enacted at the state level. Although laws regulating smoking for health reasons are largely a phenomenon of the past 10 years, cigarette smoking has been the subject of restrictive legislation for nearly a century. Early legislation had two different purposes. The first rational, relatively noncontroversial reason was the protection of the public from fire or other safety hazards, largely in the workplace. The more controversial second reason stemmed from a moral crusade against cigarettes, similar in tone and coincident with the moral crusade against alcohol that emerged in the early 1900s. Its goal was a total ban on cigarettes, which were blamed for social evils and physical ills based largely on unfounded claims. The movement lost momentum when enforcement of regulations proved controversial and difficult; all state laws banning smoking were repealed in 1927, as part of the strong reaction to alcohol prohibition.

During the 1960s, as health risks of smoking became more recognized, public policy on smoking began to focus on encouraging smokers to quit. In the early 1970s, new laws on smoking were enacted, and for the first time were extended to privately owned facilities. The laws had more restrictive language, and stated their intent to promote the safety and comfort of nonsmokers. Table 3-1 summarizes the history and extent of the laws regulating smoking in public places and worksites in the United States.

FEDERAL REGULATIONS CONCERNING SMOKING

Workplace Smoking Policies

Three federal agencies administer 90% of federal office space: The General Services Administration (GSA), the Department

(Text continued on p. 100)

Table 3-1
State Laws Regulating Smoking in Public Places and Worksites (1)

State Year(s) Legislation Enacted	AL —	AK 1975 1984	AZ 1973 1981	AR 1977 1985	CA 1971 1976 1980 1981 1982	CO 1977 1985(1)	CT 1973 1974 1983
PUBLIC PLACES WHERE SMOKING IS PROHIBITED (EXCEPT IN DESIGNATED AREAS)							
Public transportation		X	X	(X)(2)	X(3,4)	X	X(3)
Elevators		X(5)	X			X	X(5)
Indoor recreational or cultural facilities (6)		X	X		X	X	
Retail stores		(X)(7)			(X)(7)	X	X
Restaurants		X(8)			X(9)	X	X(10)
Schools		X	X	X	X	X	X
Health care facilities:							
Hospitals		X	X	X	X	X	X
Nursing homes		X			X	X	X
Public meeting rooms		X			X		X
Libraries		X	X				
Restrooms		X(5)	X			X	X
Waiting rooms		X	X			X	X
Other		X(26,27)	x)27)				
WORKSITE SMOKING RESTRICTIONS (16)							
Public worksites		D(17)			B	D(1)	B
Private worksites		A					B
IMPLEMENTATION PROVISIONS							
Nonsmokers prevail in disputes		X					
No discrimination against nonsmokers							
ENFORCEMENT							
Penalties for violations		X	X	X	X		X
Smoking		X(23d)	X(23p)	X(23e)	X(23e)		X(23c)
Failure to post signs		X(24h)					
Overall State law restrictiveness: (25)	0	3	2	1	3	3	4

(1) Executive order.
(2) School buses only.
(3) Including school buses.
(4) California stipulates that at least 50% of all passenger seats must be in nonsmoking areas on trains, airplanes, and street railroad cars departing from the State.
(5) Smoking never permitted in this area.

DE 1960	DC 1979	FL 1983 1985	GA 1975	HI 1976	ID 1925 1975 1985	IL	IN	IA 1978	KS 1975	KY 1972
X	X	X(3,5)	X(5)		X			X	X	X
	X	X(5)	X(5)	X	X			X	X	
		X		X	X			X	X	
	X	X			X					
		X(8)			X					
	X	X			X					X
	X	X		X	X			X	X	
	X	X			X			X	X	
	X	X		X	X			X	X	
		X						X	X	
		X								
		X		X						
		X(26,27,30)								
	B	B,D(18)		B(1)	B			D		
		B,D								
X	X	X	X	X	X			X	X	X
X(23c)	X(23e)	X(24i)	X(23e)	X(23e)	X(23d)			X(23e)	X(23c)	X(23a)
	X(24h)									
1	2	4	1	2	3	0	0	2	2	1

(6) Indoor recreational and cultural facilities: museums, auditoriums, theaters, and sports arenas.
(7) Grocery stores only.
(8) Restaurants seating 50 or more persons must have a no-smoking section.
(9) Restaurants seating 50 or more persons must have a no-smoking section if the restaurant is in a publicly owned building.
(10) Restaurants seating 75 or more persons must have a no-smoking section.

Table 3-1 (continued)
State Laws Regulating Smoking in Public Places and Worksites (1)

State Year(s) Legislation Enacted	LA	ME 1954 1981 1983 1985	MD 1957 1975	MA 1924 1947 1975	MI 1967 1968 1978	MN 1971 1975	MS 1942
	—						
PUBLIC PLACES WHERE SMOKING IS PROHIBITED (EXCEPT IN DESIGNATED AREAS)							
Public transportation		X	X	X(5)	(X)(2)	X	X
Elevators			X	X(5)	X	X	
Indoor recreational or cultural facilities (6)				X		X	
Retail stores		X		(X)(7)	X	X	
Restaurants					X	X(11)	
Schools						X	
Health care facilities:							
Hospitals		X	X	X	X	X	
Nursing homes		X	X	X	X	X	
Public meeting rooms						X	
Libraries				X		X	
Restrooms		X				X	
Waiting rooms		X				X	
Other		X(26)		X(26)		X(26,27)	
WORKSITE SMOKING RESTRICTIONS (16)							
Public worksites		B,D				D(17)	
Private worksites		B,D				D(17,21)	
IMPLEMENTATION PROVISIONS							
Nonsmokers prevail in disputes						X	
No discrimination against nonsmokers		X					
ENFORCEMENT							
Penalties for violations		X	X	X	X	X	X
Smoking		X(23d)	X(23h)	X(23j)	X(23k)	X(23n)	X(23o)
Failure to post signs		X(24e)			X(24e)		
Overall State law restrictiveness: (25)	0	4	2	2	3	4	1

(11) Restaurants must designate at least 30% of their seats as a no-smoking area.
(12) Restaurants are encouraged to establish no-smoking areas.
(13) Restaurants must designate at least 50% of their seats a no-smoking area.
(14) (Deleted)
(15) No place other than a bar may be designated a smoking area in its entirety.
(16) Worksite (only B, C, and D count as having a worksite policy in calculation of totals): A—Employer must post a sign prohibiting smoking at the worksite;

MO —	MT 1979	NE 1979	NV 1911 1975	NH 1981	NJ 1955 1979 1985	NM 1985	NY 1921 1975 1976	NC —	ND 1977	OH 1981 1984
	X	X	X	X	X	X	X		X	X
	X	X	X	X	X	X			X	X
	X	X	X	X	X	X	X		X	X
	X	X		X	X					
	X	X			X(12)	X(13)			X	
	X	X	X	X	X	X			X	X
	X	X	X	X	X	X			X	X
	X	X	X	X	X	X			X	X
	X	X	X	X	X	X			X	X
		X	X		X	X	X		X	X
		X							X	X
		X	X	X					X	X
		X(27)		X(29)			X(29)			
	D(19)	D(17)		D(20)	B,C(17)	B,C(20)			C	C
	D(19)	D(17,21)	A(22)		B,C(17)		A(22)			
					X					
	X	X	X	X	X	X	X		X	X
		X(23e)	X(23e)	X(23l)	X(23g)	X(23c)	X(23e)		X(23c)	X(23m)
	X(24c)				X(24g)					
0	4	4	2	2	4	3	2	0	3	2

B—Employer must have a (written) smoking policy; C—Employer must have policy that provides a nonsmoking area; D—No smoking except in designated areas.

(17) Employer must post signs designating smoking and no-smoking areas.

(18) Employer must post signs in smoking areas.

(19) Employer must post either smoking or no-smoking signs, depending upon their policy.

Table 3-1 (continued)
State Laws Regulating Smoking in Public Places and Worksites (1)

State Year(s) Legislation Enacted	OK 1975	OR 1973 1975 1977 1981	PA 1927 1947 1977	RI 1976 1977	SC 1937	SD 1974
PUBLIC PLACES WHERE SMOKING IS PROHIBITED (EXCEPT IN DESIGNATED AREAS)						
Public transportation	X			X	(X)(2)	X
Elevators	X	X		X		X
Indoor recreational or cultural facilities (6)	X	X	X	X		X
Retail stores		X	X	X		
Restaurants		X		X		
Schools		X		X		X
Health care facilities:						
Hospitals		X	X	X		X
Nursing homes		X	X	X		
Public meeting rooms		X				
Libraries	X			X		X
Restrooms						
Waiting rooms		X				
Other			X(30)	X(28)		
WORKSITE SMOKING RESTRICTIONS (16)						
Public worksites		D				
Private worksites						
IMPLEMENTATION PROVISIONS						
Nonsmokers prevail in disputes						
No discrimination against nonsmokers						
ENFORCEMENT						
Penalties for violations	X	X	X	X		X
Smoking	X(23e)	X(23b)	X(23c)	X(23e)		X(23p)
Failure to post signs		X(24e)		X(24e)		
Overall State law restrictiveness: (25)	2	3	2	3	1	2

(20) Employer must post signs in no-smoking areas.

(21) State does not restrict smoking in factories, warehouses, and similar places of work not usually frequented by the general public.

(22) Prohibits smoking in any mill or factory in which a no-smoking sign is posted.

(23) Persons who smoke in a prohibited area are subject to a fine or a penalty. Maximum fines or penalties, where applicable, are listed below: a = \$5; b = \$10; C = \$25; d = \$50; e =\$100; f = \$100/day; g = \$200; h = \$300; i = \$500; j = \$50

TX 1975	UT 1976 1979	VT 1892	VA	WA 1983	WV 1913 1919 1985	WI 1984	WY	Total N (%) 51 (100)
X	X			X(5)	X	X		35 (68.6)
X	X			X(5)		X		31 (60.8)
X	X			X(5)		X		29 (59.6)
	X			X(5)		X		18 (35.3)
	X			X		X		18 (35.3)
X	X			X(5)	X	X		27 (52.9)
X	X			X		X		33 (64.7)
X	X			X		X		29 (56.9)
	X			X(5)				21 (41.2)
X	X			X				19 (37.2)
				X				11 (21.6)
				X		X		16 (31.4)
				X(15)				12 (23.5)
	D(17)			D		D(18)		22 (43.1)
	D(17,22)	A(22)		D	A(22)			9 (17.6)
	X							4 (7.8)
	X							2 (3.9)
X	X	X		X	X	X		40 (78.4)
X(23a)	X(23a)	X(23a)		X(23f)	X(23a)	X(23c)		39 (76.5)
					X(24e)			9 (17.6)
2	4	1	0	4	1	3	0	

or up to 10 days in jail or both; k = $50 or 90 days imprisonment; l = civil action; m = minor misdemeanor; n = petty misdemeanor; o = misdemeanor; p = petty offense.

(24) Persons who are required to and fail to post smoking and/or no-smoking signs are subjected to a penalty. Maximum fines, where applicable, are listed in footnote 23.

Footnotes (continued)
(25) Restrictiveness key: 0 = None, no statewide restrictions; 1 = Nominal, State regulates smoking in one to three public places, excluding restaurants and private worksites; 2 = Basic, State regulates smoking in four or more public places, excluding restaurants and private worksites; 3 = Moderate, State regulates smoking in restaurants but not private worksites; 4 = Extensive, State regulates smoking in private worksites.
(26) Jury rooms.
(27) Halls and stairs.
(28) Stables.
(29) Polling places.
(30) Prisons, at prison official's discretion.

of Defense (DoD), and the Postal Service. In addition, the Veterans Administration (VA) develops policies for VA hospitals and clinics across the country. Over 2 million civilian federal workers and 2 million military personnel are affected by the policies of these agencies. Some agency-wide workplace smoking policies date back to 1973 or earlier, but most have been enacted or revised more recently. In general, revisions have made policies more restrictive of workplace smoking and have explicitly considered the protection of nonsmokers. Each of the current policies handles smoking in work areas differently, ranging from requesting smokers to consider the comfort of nonsmokers to limiting smoking to designated areas.

Twelve states and more than 70 communities have passed laws regulating smoking in the workplace, most of them in the past four years. Some laws apply only to public workplaces and some to both public and private workplaces. Two provisions are common to many of the state laws: restricting smoking to designated areas and requiring signs to define smoking and nonsmoking areas. Employers are given leeway in designating smoking areas. Most states rely on employers' compliance with the law's intent to provide a healthful environment; two state laws stipulate that the nonsmokers' preferences take precedence in determining work area smoking policies.

Smoking policies in the private sector have shifted in emphasis during the past five years. Previous concern centered mainly on the protection of workers and property against cigarette caused fires, on product purity, and on the protection of equipment. Today, protection of nonsmokers and regulations requiring smoking policies are the forces behind most policies in the private sector. According to recent surveys, approximately 30% of all workplaces have formal smoking policies, and there appears to be a trend toward increasing adoption of policies in the private sector. The most prevalent type of policy is one that restricts smoking in certain areas such as auditoriums, elevators, and conference rooms. Some businesses allow smoking only in specially designated areas. A few companies have recently banned smoking entirely from the workplace, and a small number hire only nonsmokers.

SMOKING REGULATIONS IN SPECIFIC PUBLIC AREAS

Public Transportation

Because high concentrations of environmental tobacco smoke can and do accumulate inside publicly used vehicles, smoking is usually restricted in such vehicles. Smoking is usually banned entirely in vehicles where riders spend little time, and confined to special areas where persons spend several hours. Such restrictions pose little problem for most persons. Smoking on interstate transport vehicles, such as buses, trains, and planes, is regulated by federal agencies.

Retail Stores

State and local legislation prohibits smoking in stores; 18 states currently prohibit such smoking. Proprietors and trade associations have supported nonsmoking restrictions because of the cost of damage to facilities and merchandise from cigarette burns.

Restaurants

According to National Restaurant Association statistics, the average American eats out 3.7 times per week; this creates the potential for repeated exposure to environmental tobacco smoke. Small restaurants have a greater problem than large facilities, because ventilation may not be able to remove smoke efficiently and room size may prevent a separation between smokers and nonsmokers. Public opinion has supported restrictions that would separate smokers from nonsmokers in restaurants; in a 1983 poll, 91% of nonsmokers and 86% of smokers supported restricting or banning restaurant smoking, with most preferring restriction. Smoking regulations in restaurants have developed through private initiative and public mandate.

In 1974, Connecticut was the first state to require restaurants to have nonsmoking sections; by 1980, 8 other states followed. At the present, 18 states have laws to regulate smoking in restaurants, and a vast number of localities regulate such smoking. Bars that do not serve meals are not included in the regulations.

There has been more opposition to smoking restrictions in restaurants than in other privately owned public places; opposition has been mainly from restaurant associations, and has been concerned with government intrusion into business practice, practical problems in the seating of smoker and nonsmokers, and the loss of the business of smokers who choose not to wait for seating in restricted areas.

Hotels and Motels

Smoking restriction in hotels and motels are private initiatives, introduced by management in response to customer demand. Hotel and motel rooms are not covered by state and local regulations and have not been addressed by nonsmoker rights advocates. Designation of rooms as nonsmoking began in the 1970s, and at the present, most large chains have some policy of this type. Designation of rooms as nonsmoking gives patrons a chance to avoid stale tobacco odors; it is not known if they can thus avoid environmental tobacco smoke. Regulation of smoking in these establishments is supported by public opinion. Hotels and motels regard the nonsmoking option as a marketing tool.

Schools

State legislation, state and local school board regulations, and individual school policies regulate smoking by students in schools. (Colleges and universities are not discussed here.) Smoking in schools has been traditionally restricted to prevent adolescents from beginning the smoking habit, or from gaining the implied approval of the habit. Teacher smoking is also regulated by many school boards. In 27 states, schools are among the public areas where smoking is restricted to designated places. In 35 states, the sale or use of tobacco by minors is prohibited; these laws provide a legal incentive for schools to regulate student smoking. For teachers and staff, the school is the workplace, with potential for environmental tobacco smoke exposure; for students, the school is the site where they spend the most time away from home. Total prohibition of smoking on school grounds provides the greatest protection from sidestream smoke exposure.

Health Care Facilities

Restrictions on smoking in health care facilities are very important; many patients treated in these facilities have illnesses which are worsened by exposure to tobacco smoke. Hospitals convey messages about health to patients and visitors; permitting smoking on these premises undermines that message. Public opinion favors restricting smoking at health care facilities. Guidelines for implementing hospital smoking policies are available.

CURRENT STATUS OF SMOKING REGULATIONS IN THE WORKPLACE

Policies regulating smoking in the workplace for worker health protection are new as of the 1980s. As of 1986, smoking is restricted or banned in 35%–40% of private businesses and in an increasing number of federal, state, and local government offices. Private sector smoking is regulated by law in 9 states and in over 70 local areas. Actions to restrict or ban smoking in the workplace are supported by a large majority of both smokers and nonsmokers.

The restriction of workplace smoking has become a major point in health concerns, because urban adults spend more time at work than at any other location except home. For adults living in a nonsmoking home, workplace exposure is the greatest source of ETS exposure. This workplace exposure is of particular concern to those individuals who are also exposed to toxic materials during the course of their work, and the effects of these toxins may be synergistic with ETS. In the workplace, individuals have less choice about ETS exposure than they do in restaurants or other public areas.

The nonsmoker's right to clean air in the workplace is supported by common law precedent; clean air at work has received much attention recently from policymakers and nonsmokers' rights advocates. Behavioral scientists have attempted to use the interpersonal relationships present in the workplace to assure the success of smoking cessation programs. Workplace smoking habits may cause employees to begin smoking; many blue-collar workers have reported that their smoking habits began when they started their jobs.

Smoking Policies

Legislation mandating smoking policies in the private sector workplace has not made as much progress as that covering public places. Private employers have been reluctant to impose behavior rules not directly related to employment. The concept of workplace smoking restriction has become more acceptable to employers and legislators as the hazards of involuntary smoking have become more widely understood, and as the attitudes about public smoking have changed. The rationale for enforcement of nonsmoking policies has arisen as a guarantee of employee right to a healthy work environment.

Prevalence of Smoking Policies

A long noncontroversial tradition of restricting smoking in the workplace exists to insure the safety of the worker, workplace, and product. Employers have restricted smoking to prevent fires or explosions around flammable materials, or to prevent product contamination. These policies date back to 1892, when Vermont authorized employers to ban smoking in factories as long as signs were posted. New York, Nevada, and West Virginia enacted similar laws, and in 1924, smoking in stables was banned because of the fire hazard.

Restrictions remained rare during the 1960s; however, during the 1970s, workplace smoking regulations were included in comprehensive clean indoor air legislation being considered at the state level. In 1975, Minnesota became the first state to enact regulations for private workplaces to protect employee health. Since that time, eight other states have enacted legislation of this type. The scope of the legislative effort widened in the 1980s to include local government; this has been strongest in California, where ordinances in 66 communities cover 44% of the state's population.

Workplace smoking regulations remained limited during the 1970s; the rules that were in place applied primarily to blue-collar areas, and were motivated by safety considerations. Policies were common in industries where there were product safety concerns, such as in the food or pharmaceutical industries, or where there might be explosion hazards. Adverse impact on clients as well as on products were given by some firms during the 1970s as reasons for implementing smoking regulations. The impact of smoking on the health of the employer as well as the employee was not mentioned. Fewer than 1% of employers polled had determined the costs of employee smoking.

Surveys made during those years, of firms that had smoking restrictions, showed that restrictions were moderate, worksite cessation programs uncommon, and nonsmoking incentives rare. Outright smoking bans were not mentioned. However, employee smoking complaints were noted by about one-third of firms polled. Five years later, the picture had changed. Firms polled in the next five years showed workplace smoking restrictions to be in place at about 35% to 55% of the firms, more firms had adopted policies which reflected the 1980s thinking about smoking, and an increasing number of firms were considering adoption of such regulations.

The nature and scope of the regulations and restrictions changed during the 1980s; the most common policy that was reported restricted smoking to specific places, total bans were still rare, and hiring preferences for nonsmokers were increasing. Workplace cessation programs increased, but nonsmoking incentives were still rare. At this writing, workplace smoking policies are nonuniform, are slightly more prevalent in large firms than in small ones, and policies are more prevalent in nonmanufacturing firms than in blue-collar businesses.

Reasons for Adopting Smoking Policies

The most often cited reasons for workplace smoking restrictions are the health protection of the employee, especially the nonsmoker, and to assure the safety of the working environment. A third reason given is compliance with state and local statutes mandating workplace smoking regulations, and a fourth reason given is to anticipate or handle demands by nonsmoking employees for a smoke-free working environment. Economic considerations, such as the loss of worktime for employee smoking breaks, are cited by some firms as reasons for not having certain types of smoking policies. Many firms do not see workplace smoking policies as being related to health insurance costs, and economic reasons do not appear to influence the promotion of workplace smoking policies.

Barriers to the Adoption of Smoking Policies

Worker discontent, cost of implementation, unacceptable policy to employees, and no employee smoking complaints are reasons given by firms not wishing to adopt workplace smoking regulations. Fear of worker discontent, or union disapproval, are also given by such firms. Other firms stated that management implements such policies without input from workers or unions. The AFL-CIO Executive Council stated its opposition to such policies and encourages the resolution of conflicts on a case-by-case basis. Other firms that have not established policies report that implementation would be difficult and rules nonenforceable. Some of these firms do business with tobacco-related companies, and do not wish to jeopardize this relationship.

Types of Smoking Policies

Private sector businesses have addressed employee smoking issues in various ways. In addition to smoking policies, the concept of "worksite smoking control" can include campaigns to educate workers to quit, self-help programs, organized smoking treatment programs, medical advice, and nonsmoking incentives. Smoking programs are often included in corporate health programs.

Businesses have taken a variety of approaches to workplace smoking policies; the choices reflect the firms motives in adopting the policies and their enforceability. Such choices depend on the goals of the policies; if employee safety is a consideration, the policies will be aimed at blue-collar workers; if the goal is to avoid customer dislike of smoking, then the policies will be aimed at customer contact situations.

Because smoke travels, it is difficult to take into consideration both smokers and nonsmokers. Firms wishing to preserve employee relationships will go to great lengths to preserve the smokers' rights by installing elaborate ventilation systems, or may separate smokers from nonsmokers. Total smoking bans will be utilized by firms that have determined that smoking is a hazard, for safety or health reasons. Cost-conscious firms will choose methods that do not involve expensive structural changes and, therefore, may choose methods that involve behavior modification to encourage smokers to quit. Total workplace smoking bans, or the hiring of only nonsmokers will be more the likely choices of firms which decide to use the latter methods. Adopting no policy at all may be a cost-effective method, if there are no employee conflicts over smoking.

To summarize current smoking plans, the following list is offered:

1. No explicit policy (the "individual solution" approach)
2. Environmental alterations (separating smokers by using physical barriers or air filters, or altering ventilation)
3. Restricting employee smoking:
    a. smoking permitted except in designated no-smoking areas
    b. smoking prohibited except in designated areas
4. Banning all workplace smoking
5. Preferential hiring of nonsmokers

1. The "Individual Solution" Approach to Workplace Smoking

Having no explicit smoking policy is still the most prevalent approach to workplace smoking; smokers and nonsmokers work out differences by themselves using common courtesy or some other approach. According to some surveys, about 70% of firms have used this approach. When there is no explicit policy, the implicit message is that there is no harm or hazard in workplace smoking. However, there is a growing consensus, even among smokers, that favors abstention in the presence of nonsmokers and a workplace smoking policy that restricts smoking.

2. Environmental Alterations

Alterations to the workplace environment range from separating smokers from nonsmokers to installing special ventilating systems to remove tobacco smoke. This latter approach involves no behavioral modifications for smokers and pleases nonsmokers. However, tobacco smoke diffuses beyond simple physical boundaries, providing only a slight reduction in exposure; and ventilation systems are expensive and may not be able to clean the air completely. Workplace modification may be the first step toward more restrictive smoking policies.

3. Restrictions on Employee Smoking

Restrictions on where employees may smoke is the most common form of workplace smoking policy and has broad public support. Policies differ on the proportion of the workplace in which smoking is allowed; whether the default condition is smoking, nonsmoking, or unspecified; who has the authority to designate the smoking status of an area; and whose wishes prevail when smokers and nonsmokers disagree. Policies often categorize worksites into four areas that are subject to different rules: private offices, shared work areas, common use areas, and large common use areas such as meeting rooms or cafeterias.

The least restrictive policies permit smoking except in certain areas, indicating that smoking is the company norm. Authority to designate these areas and the wishes of nonsmokers vs. smokers may not be clear-cut. The usual pattern is for common use areas to be designated as totally nonsmoking or partly nonsmoking. Private areas are at the discretion of the occupants. In shared office areas, compromise or individual authority for part of the area are the norm. Sidestream smoke is still a problem in shared areas.

The most restrictive smoking policies are those that specify that smoking is prohibited except in designated spaces, establishing nonsmoking as the company norm. In the strictest policies, smoking is prohibited in shared work areas, unless all area users agree to designate the area as smoking permitted; and common use areas do not permit smoking. Stricter policies stipulate both location and time when smoking is permitted, such as smoking on work breaks only. As long as the smoking areas do not contaminate the remainder of the workplace air, these policies provide greater protection of workers from side-stream smoke at the cost of greater inconvenience to smokers. Smokers may perceive these policies as restrictive or coercive. Taking extra breaks to smoke may affect productivity, if smoking areas are not conveniently located to the workplace.

4. Banning Smoking in the Workplace

Outright smoking bans may be preceded over a number of years by progressively stricter smoking regulations. Smoking bans are not widely supported by public opinion and are rarely encountered; however, they are becoming more popular among large employers. Smoking bans offer the maximum protection to nonsmokers, at the cost of greater inconvenience for smokers; they send a clear message that nonsmoking is the company norm. Ventilation needs and maintenance costs due to smoking are reduced, but strict application of the policy may result in the loss of workers who smoke as well as other difficulties in enforcement. Together with smoking bans, assistance to workers wishing to quit smoking should be implemented.

5. Preferential Hiring of Nonsmokers

Preferential hiring is the most restrictive workplace smoking policy, and was virtually unthinkable some years ago. Explicit policies favoring nonsmokers are still not very common. Hiring nonsmokers ensures a smoke-free workplace and establishes that nonsmoking is the company norm. Since a non-smoking workforce should be healthier, lower health insurance premiums may also result. However, such an employment policy limits the pool of available workers, raises the question of what to do about currently employed smokers, and may cause problems with verification of smoking status. Employers may not wish to adopt a policy that restricts or compromises off-the-job activities, or makes these activities a condition of employment.

Assuring compliance with workplace smoking policies is complex; model policies usually include enforcement provisions that identify who is responsible for policy enforcement, designate penalties for noncompliance, and ensure protection of a complaining employee. Unfortunately, these provisions often are not included in workplace policies.

Implementation of Smoking Policies

Workplaces that have adopted smoking policies have had a variety of experiences in the implementation of the policies. To assist employers, the American Lung Association and the U.S. Department of Health and Human Services, Office of Disease Prevention and Health Promotion, have developed guides with recommendations on how to adopt and implement workplace smoking policies. The guides are based on the experiences of other firms.

The Bureau of National Affairs has made available a report that details the experiences of a dozen firms that considered smoking policies; case reports are included. The firms with successful policies had strong support from top management and had advisory committees that included both smokers and nonsmokers, managers, and employees. Surveys of employees are useful for assessing inconvenience and distress from involuntary smoking and the need for smoking restrictions.

The policy, once designed, must be communicated clearly and unequivocally to all employees. A written policy document should give the rationale for the policy implementation, specify where smoking will be allowed or prohibited, and define responsibility and procedures for policy enforcement and penalties for violation. Successful policies avoid criticism of smokers or setting up antagonistic situations between smokers and nonsmokers. The policies make clear the firm's intention of not requiring employees to give up smoking, but that the firm will help workers adjust to the new regulations. Giving smokers advance notice of impending policy and providing help for those who wish to quit smoking will aid in the success of the smoking policy.

Careful plans for implementing the smoking policy are needed. It is recommended that several months be allowed between the announcement of the policy and its effective date. This gives smokers time to prepare for change and to attend smoking cessation programs if they wish to quit. This also allows time for the posting of signs and the making of any structural changes necessary in the workplace.

IMPACT OF POLICIES RESTRICTING SMOKING IN PUBLIC AND IN THE WORKPLACE

Policies that regulate where smoking is permitted may have a number of indirect and direct effects. A policy that is adequately implemented and enforced will alter the behavior of smokers in no-smoking areas and should reduce the concentration of environmental tobacco smoke in those areas. There is also the potential that smoking restrictions may have broader, indirect effects on smoking behavior and on public attitudes about tobacco use.

Potential Impacts of Smoking Policies: Policy Implementation and Approval

An essential factor to be considered in evaluating the effects of a smoking policy is the degree to which the policy has been implemented as written. Successful implementation involves public awareness of the policy, compliance with the regulations, and enforcement of penalties against violations. Compliance requires not only that smokers refrain from smoking when and where prohibited from doing so, but also that decision makers develop written policies, designate nonsmoking areas, and post signs. Enforcement requires that policy violations be dealt with, either by peer action or by penalties defined within the policy. Because smoking policies are approved by the majority of persons whose behavior the policies affect, these rules are considered to be self-enforcing. When enforcement is needed, smoking policies and legislation rely primarily on peers, assuming that the nonsmoking majority of the population will enforce the policy or statute because it is in their best interest.

Nonsmokers are expected to favor smoking restrictions that offer the benefits of clean air and reduced health risks, without behavioral changes on their part. The opinions of smokers are expected to be less favorable because they expect to be inconvenienced. Some smokers welcome such a policy because they will be assured of a place to smoke legally, because they wish to quit smoking, or because of concerns about the health risks of involuntary smoking. The extent of smoker support for policies may also depend on other factors such as the amount of smoking restriction or the adequacy of policy enforcement.

Direct Effects of Smoking Policies: Air Quality and Smoking Behavior

Measures of air quality directly assess how well smoking policies meet their primary goal of the reduction of individuals' exposure to environmental tobacco smoke. Air quality also indirectly reflects the behavior of smokers and the degree of policy compliance. A direct effect of adequately implemented smoking restrictions is to limit smoking to special places, which alters the behavior of smokers in that setting.

Indirect Effects of Smoking Policies: Knowledge, Attitudes, Social Norms, and Smoking Behavior

Policies that restrict or ban smoking in public places or the workplace carry powerful messages concerning the role of tobacco smoking in society, and help to reinforce nonsmoking as the norm in behavior. Restricting smoking to protect nonsmokers may increase public knowledge of health risks of smoking and of involuntary smoking. Restrictions may also change attitudes about the social desirability of smoking and smoking in public. Changes in the knowledge or acceptance of health risks, combined with attitude shifts, contribute to changing social norms concerning smoking and where smoking is done, and whether it is an acceptable social behavior.

Changes in social norms may influence smoking behavior by reducing pressures to smoke and increasing social support for nonsmoking and cessation of smoking. The combination of changed social norms and reduced chances to smoke may encourage smokers to stop, and discourage experimentation among youth. Changing social norms may discourage teenagers and young adults who may be less inclined to experiment with a socially undesirable substance. Current smokers may be encouraged to stop smoking.

Smoking restrictions may decrease current smokers' daily cigarette consumption by reducing opportunities for smoking. By reducing the number of opportunities to smoke, cues and stimulus-response patterns that maintain smoking behavior are reduced, and relapse among ex-smokers may also be reduced. Smoking restrictions may also enable smokers to discover alternatives to smoking as a stress reduction technique.

Smoking policies may have additional impacts beyond the change in attitudes and in smoking behavior; positive economic effects may occur for employers by reversing the excess costs associated with employees who smoke. It is generally agreed that employees who smoke cost employers more than nonsmoking employees because of excess absenteeism, increased health care costs, and reduced productivity. Productivity losses to employers include maintenance costs of cigarette-related damage and refuse, and time lost due to on-the-job smoking. Annual costs of employee smoking range from $300 to $600.

Reductions in health costs depend on whether employees are encouraged to quit as a result of smoking policies. However, these reductions may not be realized for some time. There is also the possibility that employee turnover patterns or productivity will be altered by smoking policies. Costs involved in adopting smoking policies must also be considered.

Policy Evaluation: Methodology and Study Design

The evaluation of a smoking policy in a defined or restricted population, such as a cadre of employees, must take into consideration the impacts of the policy on beliefs, attitudes, and behavior of that population. The evaluation tool must also measure delayed effects of the policy.

Simultaneous assessment of outcomes in a control population strengthens confidence in the validity of the conclusions. There is always the chance that outside influences will affect the smoking behavior or workers. Longitudinal or cross-sectional sampling may be used to assess the policy outcome; longitudinal designs afford the best measure of changes in outcome, but depend on high followup rates, which may be difficult to accomplish. One-time comparisons of populations with and without policies may provide suggestions, but not conclusive data, concerning the impact of smoking policy.

Policy Evaluation: Assessing the Effects of Smoking Policies

Air quality should be measured objectively, but such measurements are costly and require special equipment. What smoke component is measured may also be subject to controversy. Air quality may also be assessed subjectively, with ratings by nonsmokers who normally occupy smoke-free areas. These assessments should be compared with ratings made prior to any smoking bans imposed by policy. Smoking behavior characteristics must be assessed to determine the influence of smoking restrictions on behavior. Public knowledge of health risks of involuntary smoking and attitudes about smoking can be assessed by surveys. Data on social norms may be inferred from survey items such as those that measure the social acceptance of smoking in public places, smoking near nonsmokers, rights of nonsmokers to clean air, prevalence of smoking, and social support for smoking cessation. Adequacy of policy implementation can be assessed by surveys that measure the knowledge of and compliance with policy. Degree of noncompliance and enforcement can be measured by observations of behavior in public places subject to smoking restrictions.

SMOKING POLICIES FOR THE FEDERAL WORKPLACE[2]

Three agencies are responsible for administering smoking policies in 90% of all Federal office space: the General Services Administration (GSA), the Department of defense (DoD), and the Postal Service. In addition, the Veterans Administration (VA) develops smoking regulations for 172 VA medical centers and 225 clinics. In the first four months of 1986, both DoD and the VA medical centers modified their smoking policies, while GSA was in the midst of policy revision. The effectiveness of these policies, or the extent to which they are implemented, which varies from office to office, were not assessed by OTA in their report. Federal employees work in a variety of settings, but policies that affect federal office workers are the subject of this report.

GENERAL SERVICES ADMINISTRATION REGULATIONS

GSA develops regulations for the buildings it manages in its role as administrator of federal property. In 1983, GSA administered 34% of all federal office space. GSA's smoking regulations are the largest single source of workplace smoking policies for civilian federal employees.

History of GSA Regulations

GSA's Public Buildings Service, responsible for the operation and maintenance of many federal office buildings, first issued smoking regulations in 1973 after reports from the Surgeon General on the dangers of smoking and after receiving requests from nonsmokers that smoking in federal buildings be restricted or prohibited. The first regulations prohibited smoking in certain common areas, such as conference rooms, auditoriums, and elevators. They also required nonsmoking areas in GSA cafeterias and limited smoking in certain medical care facilities. They encouraged, but did not require, nonsmoking areas in open office spaces. In 1976, after resistance from federal agencies, GSA permitted smoking in conference rooms if, in the opinion of the local building manager, the room was "properly ventilated." At the urging of the Department of Health, Education, and Welfare (DHEW) and the Office on Smoking and Health, GSA strengthened its regulations in 1979. Current GSA regulations are described below. In 1986, GSA was in the stages of proposing more restrictive regulations, which were to be issued after a public comment period.

Content of GSA Regulations

The intent of GSA's current workplace smoking regulations is to provide a "reasonably smoke-free environment in certain areas" of GSA-administered buildings. The regulations cite a need to control smoking in some areas "because smoke in a confined area may be irritating and annoying to nonsmokers and may create a potential hazard to those suffering from heart and respiratory diseases or allergies." In all buildings administered by GSA, smoking is prohibited in auditoriums, conference rooms, classrooms, and elevators unless excepted by the agency head. The regulations also require nonsmoking areas, designated by signs and determined by the building manager, in building cafeterias.

Smoking in open office areas, where smoke may drift into a nonsmoker's work area, is often a point of contention. GSA's regulations are less strict in open office areas than in areas such as conference rooms, although the regulations suggest that creating nonsmoking open office areas should be "thoroughly investigated" provided that "(1) efficiency of work units will not be impaired, (2) additional space will not be required, and (3) costly alterations to the space or procurement of additional office equipment will not be necessary." Workers in an office "may unanimously declare that office as a 'no-smoking' area." However, because the decision must be unanimous, smokers retain the right to reject a no-smoking policy in the work area.

Implementation of GSA Regulations

While agencies with buildings administered by GSA are required to comply with GSA workplace smoking regulations, the agencies, not GSA, are responsible for the implementation and enforcement of the regulations. There exist, therefore, a variety of conditions in federal workplaces based on the minimum requirements established by GSA. The regulations state that "nothing in these regulations precludes an agency from adopting more stringent rules in space assigned to them," and some agencies, although certainly not a majority, have adopted more stringent policies. The Agency for International Development (AID), for example, chose to limit smoking in the workplace in August, 1985 after a poll showed that 90% of its employees favored restrictions. AID's current policy stipulates that shared work areas will be nonsmoking unless unanimously declared smoking by employees in the area. This policy makes nonsmoking the norm, compared with GSA's regulations in which smoking work areas are the norm. AID officials reported few problems implementing the policy.

A complete listing of policy variations under GSA's regulations is beyond the scope of this discussion, but there are other notable examples of agencies that have adopted stricter policies. The Indian Health Service (IHS), an agency of the U.S. Public Health Service, has announced its intention to ban smoking from its health and administrative facilities. Since late 1983, the Keams Canyon IHS hospital in Arizona has been smoke-free. A large majority of major IHS facilities, 165 of 180, have banned smoking, and another 10 facilities pledged to ban smoking after September, 1986. However, in Oklahoma, a grievance has been filed by an IHS employee charging that the ban in that facility was declared without consulting the labor union. Should the grievance be upheld, IHS management would have to negotiate with the union in that facility. Region X of the Department of Health and Human Services (DHHS) in Seattle banned smoking in September, 1984 after surveying employee attitudes and consulting with its two labor unions.

DEPARTMENT OF DEFENSE POLICIES

The Department of Defense (DoD) is the largest employer in the federal workforce, employing more than 1 million civilian workers (34% of the federal civilian workforce) and over 2 million military personnel on active duty. DoD manages 31% of all federal office space.

History of DoD Smoking Policies

The Office of the Assistant Secretary of Defense for Force, Management, and Personnel developed DoD's first workplace smoking policy in 1977. Recently, the policy has been modified and incorporated into a more general health directive. The original policy prohibited smoking in certain portions of all DoD buildings, including auditoriums, conference rooms, and classrooms. It also required the establishment of nonsmoking areas in eating facilities "wherever practicable." Smoking was permitted in shared work areas "only if ventilation is adequate to remove smoke from a work area and provide an environment that is healthful." DoD defined "adequate ventilation" as at least "10 cubic feet of fresh air per minute per person." In theory, this meant that if a nonsmoker were to formally complain about smoke in his or her work area, an industrial hygienist would be called in to take measurements, the results of which might lead to a nonsmoking policy for the area. DoD's original workplace smoking policy was superseded by a more general health directive on health promotion signed by the Secretary of Defense on March 11, 1986.

Content of DoD Smoking Policies

The workplace smoking policies established in DoD's recent health directive are somewhat more stringent than the policies implemented in 1977, although the changes do not appear to be large. Smoking is prohibited in auditoriums, conference rooms, and classrooms, just as it was in 1977, and in the new directive, nonsmoking areas are required in all eating facilities rather than just "wherever practicable." The new directive also states that "smoking shall not be permitted in common work areas shared by smokers and nonsmokers unless adequate space is available for nonsmokers and ventilation is adequate to provide them a healthy environment," although "healthy environment" is not defined in the policy. The new directive also places more emphasis on smoking cessation programs than the 1977 policy did. After a recent controversy over the sale of cigarettes at reduced prices in military exchanges and commissaries, the Secretary of Defense announced DoD's intention to carry out "an intense antismoking campaign" in the military, rather than increase cigarette prices. Reduced cigarette prices were seen as part of commissary privileges, which allow military personnel to buy goods at reduced prices.

Implementation of DoD Policies

Major divisions within DoD include the Office of the Secretary of Defense, the Military Departments of the Army, Navy (which includes the Marine Corps), and Air Force, and the 12 Defense Agencies (e.g., the Defense Intelligence Agency and the Defense Mapping Agency). Each division is required to implement the health promotion directive, which includes policies on smoking in the workplace. Each of the divisions, therefore, drafts its own set of policies based on the requirements of the directive. Implementation of the policies may be stronger than the requirements set by the directive. For instance, after consulting with its labor unions, the Madigan Army Medical Center in Tacoma, Washington, banned smoking from its facilities.

POSTAL SERVICE POLICIES

The U.S. Postal Service, an independent establishment of the executive branch, employs over 700,000 workers and administers 25% of all federal office space. The Postal Service is divided into five regional areas within the United States, and among these areas there are nearly 40,000 branch offices and stations.

History of Postal Service Smoking Policies

Unlike many other federal agencies, the Postal Service has a long history of workplace smoking policies. In contrast to the policies adopted by GSA in 1973, and DoD in 1977, the Postal Service policies were issued because of the flammable nature of the mail rather than for health concerns. This consideration has been the primary impetus for smoking policies in the Postal Service, and it has been only recently that the health of nonsmoking employees has been considered a factor in determining workplace smoking policies.

Content of Postal Service Regulations

Today, the flammable nature of the mail is still the main focus of Postal Service workroom smoking policies. The regulations state that "smoking areas must be clearly designated" and that "employees must not smoke, under any circumstances, while receiving mail from the public, around belt conveyor tunnels, collecting mail from letter boxes, loading or unloading mail, distributing mail into pouches and sacks, or hanging, working, or closing pouches or sacks on racks."

These limitations apply particularly to postal workroom areas; in contrast, office smoking policies are not clearly delineated, varying from office to office. Postal regulations state that "smoking on duty is a privilege, not a right, and must not be indulged in to the detriment of the Postal Service or an employee's work, nor at the risk or discomfort of nonsmoking employees." While this reflects consideration to nonsmokers, it does not establish procedures to be followed in carrying out a policy. The Postal Service headquarters in Washington, D.C. has issued a smoking policy for its immediate office; smoking there is prohibited if a nonsmoker objects. However, this policy is presented to other offices as an example only and does not require other offices to establish similar policies.

Implementation of Postal Service Smoking Policies

To a much greater extent than other federal agencies, the Postal Service employment policies are governed by the process of collective bargaining. The Office of Safety and Health within the Postal Service has a contractual obligation to provide notice to unions and, if requested, meet with them while making policies which relate to working conditions. If a new policy were to be agreed upon, it would be printed and distributed through the *Postal Bulletin* to the five regional offices and nearly 40,000 branch offices across the country.

VETERANS ADMINISTRATION POLICIES

Two sets of policies form the basis of most Veterans Administration (VA) workplace smoking restrictions. The Department of Medicine and Surgery (DM&S) employs 190,000 (82%) of the VA's employees and administers the VA's hospitals, clinics, and nursing homes. GSA administers most of the remainder of VA buildings. GSA regulations are discussed above; this section focuses on the policies set by DM&S within the VA.

History of Veterans Administration (DM&S) Policies

The first DM&S smoking policy was written in 1978, and since then it has been revised four times. The first policy prohibited smoking in certain places, such as patient interview areas, examination areas, and conference rooms. It also stated that "where space accommodations permit," smoking and non-smoking sections should be established in areas including waiting areas, dining rooms, patient day rooms, and patient rooms. The first three policy revisions included mostly minor changes which gradually broadened the policy. The most recent revision, approved in 1986, included extensive changes.

Content of Veterans Administration (DM&S) Policies

The new DM&S policy states that "near each medical center entrance there will be a sign stating 'No smoking allowed in this medical center except in designated areas.' " Most often, specific dayrooms will be designated as smoking areas. The policy also allows smoking and nonsmoking sections in waiting areas and dining rooms, and "adequate ventilation and/or smoke eaters [mechanical devices designed to reduce smoke levels] must be provided in all designated smoking areas." Whereas patients were allowed to smoke in rooms when space allowed and the physician approved under previous policies, under the new policy, patients with physician approval "will be escorted to a designated smoking area when necessary. Those patients whose smoking would, in the judgment of an appropriate health professional, pose a risk to themselves or others, will be allowed to smoke under strict supervision only." The policy also calls for educational programs on the hazards of smoking, and smoking cessation clinics.

Implementation of Veterans Administration (DM&S) Policies

According to the 1986 policy, VA medical centers are encouraged to designate a "smoking control officer with responsibility for implementing the smoking policy at that facility." In addition, people who smoke within a nonsmoking area may be subject to a fine of up to $50, although voluntary compliance through a notification system is encouraged.

STATE AND LOCAL WORKPLACE SMOKING LAWS

An increasing number of state and local government laws have restricted smoking in the workplace, particularly since 1983. Since that time, seven state laws and more than 70 community ordinances have regulated smoking in either the public or private sectors in addition to five other states which already had such a law. OTA has complied a list of state laws regulating workplace smoking and examined a few sample local ordinances.

STATE WORKPLACE SMOKING LAWS

Minnesota was the first state to regulate smoking in the workplace with the passage of its Clean Indoor Act of 1975. Utah followed in 1976, Montana and Nebraska in 1979, and since 1981, nine other states have passed laws regulating smoking in the workplace. Rhode Island's legislation was proposed in 1986; however, Colorado, Maryland, and Virginia defeated such legislation.

State laws restrict workplace smoking in different ways; some simply require each workplace to post the policy; many others restrict smoking to designated areas only. Common to many of the laws is an explicit intention to protect the health and comfort of nonsmokers. The states with workplace smoking laws have adopted one or more of the following components.

Components of State Workplace Smoking Laws

Restricting smoking at state and local workplaces. Laws in Alaska, New Hampshire, New Mexico, and Wisconsin restrict smoking at state and local workplaces only; laws in the other states that restrict smoking in the workplace apply to both public and private workplaces. The intent of laws in the states mentioned above is to regulate smoking in "public places," which are defined from state to state to include places such as libraries and museums as well as state workplaces. Each of the laws restricts smoking to designated areas in the workplace. In Alaska, after some confusion over a provision requiring "reasonable accommodations" for the needs of smokers and nonsmokers, a state labor/management committee developed guidelines for establishing smoking and nonsmoking areas in state buildings.

Requiring a written policy. Laws passed in Connecticut, Florida, Maine, New Jersey, and New Mexico (state and local workplaces only) all require that employers establish a written smoking policy. Connecticut requires only that "each employer shall establish and post written rules governing smoking and nonsmoking in that portion of any business facility for which he is responsible." The law, which applies only to businesses with 50 or more employees in a "structurally enclosed location," does not specify the policy's intent; an employer may choose to allow smoking throughout the workplace. New Jersey's law, passed in late 1985, also specifies that businesses with 50 or more employees must establish a written policy; however, New Jersey's law also requires that employers designate nonsmoking areas. The laws in Florida and Maine are the most explicit of the five states that require employers to develop policies. In Florida, the policy "shall take into consideration the proportion of smokers and nonsmokers" and prohibit smoking except in designated areas. In Maine also, the policy "shall prohibit smoking except in designated smoking areas."

Limiting smoking to designated areas. Restricting smoking

to designated areas is a provision common to most state laws regulating smoking in the workplace. Eight states with workplace smoking laws have such a provision. Minnesota's law was the first among states to limit smoking in the workplace, stating that "no person shall smoke in a public place or at a public meeting except in designated smoking areas." Several states, including Utah, Nebraska, and Florida, followed Minnesota's example, using language from Minnesota's law to restrict smoking to designated areas. Each of these states defines "public place" to include places of work; this definition is important because other states, such as Oregon, also restrict smoking in public places; however, Oregon does not include the workplace in its definition of a "public place."

One issue raised by the language of the state laws is the definition of "designated area" for smoking. In each of the states, designation of smoking areas is left up to the person in charge of the public place within the boundaries established by the intent of the laws. Although laws in New Mexico (state and local workplaces only) and Utah are the only ones to specifically state that nonsmokers' preferences prevail over smokers' preferences, each of the above laws was written with the intention of providing a healthful work environment. Shared work areas may thereby be discouraged from being designated smoking; however, in come cases an employer may technically be in compliance with the law but in conflict with its intent by designating a shared work space as a smoking area. In Maine, the state health department considers the intent of the law as well as its technical specifications if legal action against an employer is required.

Other guidelines and constraints influence the designation of smoking areas. Negotiations with labor through collective bargaining may be required. Also, all laws except those in Alaska and Maine state that "existing physical barriers and ventilation systems" should be used to separate smoking and nonsmoking areas, eliminating a mandate for costly alterations. Laws in Minnesota, Utah, and Nebraska explicitly mention that offices occupied solely by a smoker or group of smokers may be designated as smoking areas; all the other state laws implicitly allow this.

Requiring signs to be posted. Ten states require that signs designating smoking and/or nonsmoking areas must be posted in the workplace. Alaska (state and local workplaces only), Minnesota, Nebraska, New Jersey, and Utah all require signs designating smoking and nonsmoking areas. Florida and Wisconsin (state and local workplaces only) require that signs be posted in smoking areas, while laws in New Hampshire and New Mexico require signs only in nonsmoking areas in state and local workplaces. Montana's law, one of the least restrictive state laws requiring workplace smoking, requires only that a smoking or no-smoking sign be posted, depending on the policy set by the employer. Many of the laws specify a minimum size for the signs; in Minnesota, signs "shall be in printed letters of not less than 1.5 inches (3.8 centimeters) in height," unless used on a table or seat.

Giving preference to nonsmokers in resolving conflicts. In New Mexico, in state and local offices occupied by smokers and nonsmokers, the employer must provide a smoke-free work area to accommodate any employee who requests one, as long as costly modifications are not required. And Utah's law, which limits smoking to designated areas, requires employers to comply by allowing an employee who is in an individual work area to make his work area smoke-free, as long as it is posted as such. The employer in Utah must give this nonsmoking employee precedence over a smoker in resolving agreements concerned with workplace smoking. Although Minnesota's law does not have a clause explicitly giving preference to nonsmokers, state health officials interpret the law's intent and its sections on designation of smoking areas as giving precedence to nonsmokers' concerns.

Prohibiting action against nonsmokers who complain about smoking. Two state laws explicitly prohibit taking action against nonsmokers because they complain about smoking. In Utah, an employer is not allowed to "discriminate against an employee who expresses concern about smoke pollution in the place of employment which is detrimental to his health or comfort.'' And in Maine, ''it is unlawful for any employer to discharge, discipline, or otherwise discriminate against any of its employees because that employee has assisted in the supervision or enforcement of this section.''

Enforcement of State Laws

States have various provisions for enforcement of laws regulating workplace smoking, but in general, the laws tend to be self-enforcing. In nearly all states, the state health department or its local subdivision is responsible for enforcement of the law. Some states, such as Connecticut and New Jersey, essentially have no provisions for enforcement or penalties, while others, Utah and Florida in particular, may assess fines up to $299 or $500, respectively, for violation of the law, although in practice such high fines have never been assessed. In seven of the states, a smoker can be cited for a non-criminal violation or charged for a misdemeanor if found smoking in a nonsmoking area. Also, in seven of the states, an employer who fails to implement provisions of the law may also be held responsible, either through fines, a court injunction, or misdemeanor conviction.

In telephone conversations with state employees responsible for implementing the laws, OTA found that most of their effort was spent during the phase-in period when employers were uncertain about compliance standards. States which have had workplace smoking policies for a few years reported few enforcement problems. Utah's law has been in effect since 1976, and the state officials responsible for enforcement estimated that in recent years, about six employers had been fined from $25 to $50.

LOCAL WORKPLACE SMOKING ORDINANCES

More than 70 communities in California have passed ordinances regulating smoking in the workplace. California has been by far the most active state, but communities in other states, including New York, Ohio, and Colorado have also passed workplace smoking ordinances. Local workplace smoking ordinances are a recent and rapidly-developing phenomenon; nearly all have been written since 1983, and in the first two months of 1986, Nassau County in New York adopted, and New York City's Mayor Koch proposed, workplace smoking ordinances.

City Ordinances

The most active state in passing workplace smoking ordinances at the city level has been California. After nonsmokers' legislation was defeated twice at the state level, groups such as the Californians for Non-smokers Rights shifted their emphasis to ordinances at the local level.

In 1983, 13 California cities passed nonsmoking ordinances, including San Francisco and Palo Alto. In San Francisco, each employer must establish an office smoking policy. San Francisco's workplace smoking ordinance states that "if an employer allows employees to smoke in the workplace, then this ordinance requires (1) that the employer make accommodations for the preferences of both nonsmoking and smoking employees, and (2) if a satisfactory accommodation to all affected nonsmoking employees cannot be reached, that the employer prohibit smoking in the office workplace." The ordinance does not apply to enclosed offices occupied solely by smokers, state or Federal government buildings, or homes that serve as workplaces. The ordinance is enforced with a fine of up to $500 for any employer who fails to comply; however, few problems with enforcement have been reported.

Palo Alto's ordinance, passed in 1983 after San Francisco's ordinance, goes a step further by allowing a worker to declare his or her work area as nonsmoking. According to the ordinance, "any employee in the office workplace shall be given the right to designate his or her immediate area as a nonsmoking area and to post it with appropriate signs or sign." The ordinance goes on to state that "in any dispute arising under the smoking policy, the rights of the nonsmoker shall be given precedence.'' As with the San Francisco ordinance, Palo Alto's ordinance does not apply to enclosed offices occupied solely by smokers, to state or Federal office buildings, or to private homes that serve as a workplace. Violation of the ordinances is an infraction of city code; fines range form $50 to $250.

As of March 1986, 67 cities and towns and 7 counties in California have ordinances regulating smoking in the workplace. Across the state, 44% of the population falls under the jurisdiction of a local workplace smoking ordinance. For some companies with statewide offices, complying with the variety of ordinances in different cities has been something of a problem; the Pacific Telesis company in California developed a flexible corporate smoking policy in response to the situation.

County Ordinances

In 1984, Suffolk County in New York State adopted a workplace smoking ordinance for offices of 50 or more employees, similar in many ways to Palo Alto's city ordinance. According to the Suffolk ordinance, ''any employee in the office workplace shall be given the right to designate his or her immediate area as a nonsmoking area and to post it with an appropriate sign or signs.'' However, unlike Palo Alto's ordinance, it adds that ''in any dispute arising under the smoking policy, the rights of the nonsmoker shall be governed by the rule of reason and economic practicability of action by the employer.'' The ordinance also prohibits smoking in many areas where both smokers and nonsmokers might be present, including conference rooms, auditoriums, restrooms, and elevators. The maximum fine for violation of the ordinance is $25.

Nassau County, a neighboring county to Suffolk in New York State, passed a smoking ordinance in 1986 that limits smoking in the workplace to designated areas. Cited as ''among the toughest in the country,'' the ordinance bans smoking in many public places including hospitals, movie theaters, and stores, and prohibits smoking in specific areas of the workplace, such as in cafeterias, conference rooms, restrooms, and work areas. The ordinance states, however, that "an employer may designate a separate portion or portions of the work area, employees' lounge, and cafeteria, for smoking." Designating open work areas as smoking areas is discouraged by the County Board of Health if it conflicts with the intent of the ordinance "to provide [county] residents protection from exposure to tobacco smoke." The ordinance is enforced by fines of up to $500; two full-time administrators were assigned to administer the ordinance during phase-in.

WORKPLACE SMOKING POLICIES IN THE PRIVATE SECTOR

Private sector smoking policies have shifted emphasis and increased in number in the last few years. In that time, nonsmokers' rights groups pressed for increased restriction of smoking in the workplace. Workplace smoking policies today are more likely to be based on consideration of the health and comfort of nonsmokers than policies four or five years ago that tended to emphasize the protection of products and equipment and the prevention of fires and explosions.

Employer decisions to implement smoking policies are undoubtedly motivated by a number of factors, including concern for employee health and the costs of ill health, compliance with state and local laws, and a desire to reduce potential sources of conflict between employees. Employers may also wish to reduce their potential liability from lawsuits, and worker's compensation, unemployment benefits, and disability benefit claims by passively exposed nonsmokers. However, the extent of this potential liability is currently unclear and is probably only a subsidiary motivation.

Smoking Policy Surveys

Survey data indicate that in 1980, most existing workplace policies were written with the intent to protect products and equipment in the workplace, to accommodate customers and clients, or to restrict smoking in blue-collar work areas for reasons of workers' safety. Examples of these types of policies include smoking restrictions in food processing industries and bank lobbies and restrictions imposed to prevent fires and explosions.

Recent surveys of workplace smoking policies have been conducted by the Office of Disease Prevention and Health Promotion (ODPHP) in the Department of Health and Human Services, and by a California consulting firm funded by the Tobacco Institute. The ODPHP survey data were scheduled for release in July 1986. The survey polled over 1600 worksites with 50 or more employees nationwide on health promotion activities in the workplace, with a response rate of about 85%. The survey differs from previous surveys in that the sample consists of actual worksites defined by location, as opposed to central company offices. The survey conducted for the Tobacco Institute polled 1100 large firms and had a response rate of 40%. The firms chosen for the Tobacco Institute survey were drawn from the *Fortune* 1000 service and industrial companies and *Inc.* magazines's 100 fastest growing companies.

Both surveys, though based on very different samples of workplaces, produced similar estimates of the prevalence of workplace smoking policies. The ODPHP survey found that 36% of worksites with 750 or more employees had smoking policies, while the Tobacco Institute survey found that 32% of large firms surveyed had a smoking policy.

One conclusion drawn in the Tobacco Institute study, that "workplace smoking policies are not a trend among major companies," does not appear to be supported by their data. The survey inidcates that 9% of the firms with smoking policies had developed them in the year before the survey, and 20% in the previous five years. These data should be interpreted cautiously, however, as nearly 60% of those responding did not know how long the policy had been in effect.

Results from the ODPHP survey indicate that nonsmokers' concerns and regulations requiring smoking policies have become primary reasons for workplace smoking policies. Results suggest that 27% of all worksites with 50 or more employees have some form of smoking policy, and that the primary purpose of 40% of these policies was to "protect nonsmokers." Another 40% were written to "comply with regulations," and 13% of the policies were written to "protect equipment." The primary purpose for 7% of the policies was "to protect high risk employees," such as asbestos workers.

Private Sector Smoking Restrictions

Private sector businesses demonstrate a variety of approaches for accommodating nonsmokers' concerns. Although this report focuses on policies, it should be mentioned that many private sector businesses also use smoking cessation programs and incentives to help employees quit smoking in conjunction with the policies. The most widely used cessation programs, according to the ODPHP survey, are self-help program materials to be used on the smoker's own time. These include information packets and videotapes from sources such as the American Lung Association. Some businesses offer financial incentives such as bonuses for smoking abstinence.

It is not always possible to neatly categorize the motives and expectations behind specific private sector policies. Private sector workplace smoking policies range from policies concerned primarily with occupational safety and product purity, to a growing number of policies concerned with nonsmokers' health and comfort. Some industries, such as the health and insurance industries, are especially inclined to restrict smoking for health reasons. The airline industry is required by federal regulations to establish smoking and nonsmoking sections on all large aircraft and to prohibit smoking on aircraft with less than 30 seats.

In this section, OTA focused on workplaces that have developed a workplace smoking policy. Data indicate that the majority of businesses do not have a policy; however, the increasing number of state and local laws regulating smoking, as well as the greater awareness of nonsmokers' concerns reflected in the ODPHP survey, suggest that the number of workplace smoking policies is increasing. OTA did not note businesses that have rescinded previous policies.

Restricting smoking in certain areas. Smoking is often banned in specific areas outside the actual work area. These policies ban smoking in areas such as meeting and conference rooms, auditoriums, elevators, bathrooms, and hallways. Although survey information is not available on the prevalence of this type of policy, it appears to be the most common type. Often, state laws or local ordinances prohibit smoking in areas such as elevators; in 1984, 40 states and the District of Columbia prohibited smoking in certain public areas. Some firms have used this type of policy as a first step in creating a more comprehensive workplace smoking policy. The Boeing Company in Seattle currently designates nonsmoking areas, but has announced its intent to ban smoking entirely.

Surveys in 1980 indicated that 54% of large Massachusetts businesses had work areas where smoking was prohibited because of potential damage to products of equipment, and smoking is often restricted in blue-collar work areas because of safety reasons. Businesses where contact with clients is frequent often restrict smoking in lobbies and other client contact areas. A 1980 survey of 500 members of the Adminstrative Management Society found that 46% of those who responded prohibited smoking in areas where employees came into contact with customers and clients, making it the most common policy among that service- and client-oriented group of firms. The policies did not restrict smoking in common work areas; rather, they prohibited it in areas where clients would be present, such as at bank teller windows. Therefore, these policies apply only to employees who normally work with clients.

Modifying the work environment. Although not so much an explicit policy or restriction as a more general means of accommodating smokers and nonsmokers, modifying the work environment is a step taken by many employers. Modifications range from posting signs to separating work areas and improving ventilation. Sometimes workplace modification is a step taken before more explicit policies are developed. In 1979, the Control Data Corporation in Minneapolis separated work areas into smoking and nonsmoking sections and designed ventilation systems to blow smoke away from nonsmokers; in 1984, Control Data banned cigarette smoking except in designated areas. One factor limiting the extent of workplace modification is cost; Minnesota's state law, for instance, requires only that "existing physical barriers and ventilation systems" be used in separating smoking and nonsmoking areas, rather than requiring new structures.

Banning smoking except in designated areas. Some firms have prohibited smoking in the workplace except in designated areas. Five states currently have laws requiring private sector employers to restrict smoking to designated areas. The Control Data Corporation in Minnesota, which has such a law, prohibits smoking in all areas except in private offices, sections of cafeterias and conference rooms, and certain refreshment rooms. MSI Insurance, also in Minnesota, limits smoking to part of the cafeteria. Some state health officials contacted by OTA had received complaints from nonsmokers in firms where smoke from designated areas drifted into the work area.

Banning smoking throughout the workplace. Recently, a small number of firms have banned smoking entirely from the workplace. Pacific Northwest Bell, based in Seattle, banned smoking late in 1985, a policy recommended by an employee committee after two years of review. The firm had also conducted a survey of employees that indicated that most employees wanted a policy regulating smoking in work areas. The Provident Indemnity Life Insurance Company in Norristown, Pennsylvania, banned smoking on company property in 1983. The firm reached that stage in steps, first by limiting smoking to the lunchroom during a certain time period, and then by altering its job application so that applicants would be aware that smokers must abide by the policy and pay for insurance at a greater rate than nonsmokers. The CIGNA Health Plan of Arizona, a health maintenance organization centered in Phoenix, banned smoking in 1985, after a resolution to make hospitals smoke free passed at a meeting of the Arizona Medical Association.

These bans seem to have been implemented smoothly, but an employer may have problems declaring a total ban if the employer declares the ban unilaterally when labor negotiations are required. In an arbitration case in California, an employer's ban was declared unreasonable by an arbitrator because it did not cite sufficient reasons for the ban and the ban had been declared unilaterally by management.

Although their numbers appear to be small, some employers also have a policy against hiring smokers. The Johns-Manville asbestos firm stopped hiring smokers in 1978, and some fire departments have recently decided to hire only nonsmokers.

SUMMARY: WORKPLACE SMOKING POLICIES

Approximately 30% of all private sector workplaces have a formal smoking policy, while a majority of Americans support smoking policies. Governments at all levels and the private sector are increasingly adopting or strengthening such policies and there is no evidence of retrenchment. In addition, the protection of nonsmokers, who account for 67% of the population, has become a primary motive for the development of policies. For these reasons, increasing adoption of more stringent workplace smoking policies will likely continue for the forseeable future.

REFERENCES

1. *Health Consequences of Involuntary Smoking: A Report of the Surgeon General.* U.S. Department of Health and Human Services, Public Health Service. Washington, DC: Superintendent of Documents, U.S. Government Printing Office, 1986. 359 pp. DHHS(CDC)87-8398. pp. 271–274.

2. *Passive Smoking in the Workplace: Selected Issues.* Staff paper prepared by the Special Projects Office of the Health Program, Office of Technology Assessment: U.S. Congress, 1986. 70 pp. (NTIS PB86-217627). pp. 1–2, 4–5, 8–59.

5

Costs and Benefits of Programs

Worksite smoking prevention programs are all too scarce in this country; only 12% of all firms with 500 or more employees have a company doctor, and only 18% of U.S. firms have a part-time physician. Company doctors usually devote their staff time to prevention of industrial disease; less than 20% of the doctor's time is spent on health education, and company nurses spend less than 25% of their time on health education. Only 58% of firms with 5000 or more workers offer any type of health education program. Smaller firms offer much less in the way of employee health education, and some offer nothing at all.

Of all possible types of industrial health education programs that are available, one of the most valuable is smoking cessation. The workplace is an ideal setting in which to provide a variety of approaches tailored to the needs of individual smokers. Large numbers of smokers are available, ongoing programs are possible, and long-term evaluation is feasible. For employees, the primary potential advantages appear to be convenience, reduced costs, and the opportunity to participate with friends and coworkers. The potential advantages to employers, discussed in previous chapters, are cost savings from reduced health insurance, reduced absenteeism, increased productivity, reduced maintenance costs, and improved employee morale.

Benefits of smoking cessation do not occur automatically; they may be offset by potential disadvantages. Programs may interfere with the work schedule, program meetings may be inconveniently scheduled, smokers may feel coerced into participating, unions may object to programs, and employers may feel burdened by program costs and lost time at work.

COSTS AND EFFECTS OF WORKPLACE SMOKING POLICIES

Any administrative or physical changes made to alter smoking behavior in the workplace are likely to generate costs and benefits, including possible cost savings and health benefits. Quantitative information from which to predict the magnitude of total costs and effects is scanty. A short discussion of some of the factors that would be included in an analysis of the costs and effects of these policies is provided in the discussion that follows, and in the OTA document mentioned in the Selected References section at the end of this book.

Cost-Effectiveness of Smoking Policies

Previous studies of the costs of smoking have focused on costs related to active smoking. Taking a society wide perspective, it has been estimated by OTA that 314,000 deaths in 1982 were attributable to smoking: 139,000 cancer deaths, 123,000 cardiovascular disease deaths, and 52,000 chronic obstructive lung disease deaths. The social costs attributable to those deaths include $12 to $35 billion in health care costs and $27 to $61 billion in lost earnings. There have also been analyses of the costs of active smoking from the perspective of both the individual and the employer.

The costs and benefits of policies concerning smoking in the workplace, however, have not been extensively analyzed. An analysis depends on both the costs of implementing the policies and on their benefits. Any analysis should also clearly identify its perspective (e.g., whether the effects arrayed are costs or benefits to society, to employers, to smokers, or to nonsmokers). In addition, while workplace smoking policies will certainly affect nonsmokers' exposures to passive smoking, these policies may also influence the extent of active smoking by smokers.

Legislation proposed by the Ninety-ninth Congress, as S. 1937, required federal agencies to issue rules designating smoking areas in U.S. government buildings. These rules would be developed in consultation with the Surgeon General and implemented after consultation with employee representatives, and were intended to "make reasonable accommodations for the needs of the smokers and nonsmokers" who use federal buildings, provide for display of signs designating smoking and no-smoking areas, and provide for enforcement of smoking prohibitions in no-smoking areas. Each of the components of this legislation would affect the degree of nonsmokers' exposures to tobacco smoke and influence the nature of the relationships between smokers and nonsmokers in the workplace.

While policies concerning smoking in the workplace seem to be successful, information on costs and effects of the policies is difficult to obtain. Because of this quantitative limitation, this report does not contain a cost-benefit or cost effectiveness analysis of workplace smoking policies. Instead, this section discusses some of the factors that would need consideration when evaluating costs and effects of these policies.

Benefits of Workplace Smoking Policies

As mentioned earlier, one recent survey indicates that a large majority of the U.S. population believes that smokers should refrain from smoking in the presence of nonsmokers, and that companies should limit smoking to designated areas. While this expressed preference would be difficult to incorporate into an economic analysis of smoking policies, it is still an important consideration in any decision concerning the creation of such policies. Another consideration is how the setting of workplace policies by the federal government will accelerate the current trends toward increased adoption of smoking policies by other levels of government and by private employers.

If workplace policies lead to reductions in exposure to passive smoking, then there should be a reduction in the incidence of smoking-related disease among nonsmokers. If treatment of these diseases requires the use of medical resources, less disease would imply savings in health care costs. Generally, reducing the incidence of nonfatal disease will lead to a saving of health care resources. Depending on the extent to which these health care costs are paid for by insurance, the saving of health care resources should lead to a reduction in the costs of health insurance.

If the diseases caused by passive smoking are fatal, prevention will result in longer life. During the additional years of life gained, additional medical resources will be used. Thus, preventing an early death may lead to savings in health care costs in the present and increases in health care costs in future years. The net effect depends on the relative costs of the diseases in question and the discount rate used in the analysis of future effects. However, analysts disagree on whether these potential future costs should be included in a cost-effectiveness analysis.

Life insurance rates will only be affected if the passive smoking-related diseases are fatal. Reducing the death rate of an insured group should lead to a reduction in the costs of providing life insurance. The extent of this reduction will depend on the size of the increase in longevity.

A few companies have restricted employment to nonsmokers in a desire to reduce the incidence of occupational disease and associated workers' compensation payments. For example, the combined effect of exposures to asbestos and cigarette smoking is much greater than the effect of exposure to only asbestos or cigarette smoke. Hiring only nonsmokers might reduce the costs of compensating workers with asbestos-related disease, although reductions in asbestos exposures represent another alternative.

Eliminating smoking from the worksite would eliminate the workplace fires started by burning cigarettes. The effect of confining smoking to designated areas is less clear. Fire prevention and control might be better if smoking is restricted to particular locations, although actions might be needed to prevent smoking in non-designated areas. The reduction in the frequency of fires and associated property damage should lead to reduction in the costs of fire losses and insurance. Of course, the magnitude of this benefit will depend on the proportion of fires associated with smoking.

Reducing workplace smoking may also lead to reductions in the costs of cleaning and maintaining the workplace. This may include reductions in the costs of cleaning offices, a lessened need to clean and repair sensitive equipment, as well as a reduction in the costs of maintaining the ventilating system (such as replacement or cleaning of filters). Reduced workplace smoking may also improve relations with customers who are irritated by tobacco smoke.

The beneficiaries of any of the reductions in insurance costs depends on the method used for financing the insurance (in particular, the relative shares of the employer and the employee). Thus, the analysis needs to be clear about who receives any particular benefit and who bears the costs of these policies.

Several sources indicate that smokers have more sick loss days than nonsmokers, although this excess may not be entirely due to smoking. If passive exposures also led to an increase in sick time, then reducing passive exposures should lead to reductions in employee absenteeism among nonsmokers.

Workplace smoking policies should also reduce or eliminate the irritation and annoyance experienced by nonsmokers when exposed to tobacco smoke. In many cases, tobacco smoke is part of the more general problem of indoor air pollution. Investigation of complaints about indoor air quality only rarely finds tobacco smoke to be the sole source of the problem. But while indoor air pollution and the "sick building syndrome" are often the result of inadequate ventilation and exposures to other toxic agents, exposure to tobacco smoke is frequently a factor in complaints of ill health associated with office work.

Thus, improving the comfort of nonsmokers and reducing tobacco smoke-induced irritation is an important benefit of these policies. Economists often suggest that the most appropriate way to place a monetary value on nonsmokers' comfort would be to estimate how much nonsmokers might be willing to pay to avoid environmental tobacco smoke. Thus, on the benefit side would be how much nonsmokers would be willing to pay to reduce or eliminate exposure to tobacco smoke; on the cost side would be estimates of how much smokers might be willing to pay to continue to smoke without restrictions. But, reliable estimates of willingness to pay are difficult to obtain and would be influenced by the income levels of the individuals affected. In addition, ethical arguments are likely to be raised. Many consider clean air to be a right and, thus, reject the idea that nonsmokers should have to pay in order to breathe clean air. Others express concern that employers and the government have no right to restrict an individual's decision to smoke.

The intended effect of smoking policies is to reduce or eliminate the exposures of nonsmokers to tobacco smoke. Another possible effect is that, faced with restrictions concerning when and where they may smoke, some smokers may reduce the amount of their smoking or give up the habit entirely. Surveys regularly report that a large majority of smokers would like to quit and that many have tried to quit. A survey at one company, Pacific Bell (now called Pacific Telesis), indicated that if a new company policy concerning smoking in the workplace was implemented, 13% of the smokers would try to quit and 38% would smoke less. Thus, even though the primary purpose of these policies is to reduce or eliminate nonsmokers' passive exposures, the implementation of workplace smoking restrictions may also motivate, encourage, or support the decisions of smokers to reduce their consumption or stop smoking entirely. Of course, if smokers quit in response to workplace smoking restrictions, their families will no longer be passively exposed, leading to additional health benefits among family members.

Costs of Workplace Smoking Policies

A number of businesses have begun workplace antismoking programs out of consideration of the costs of medical insurance for their employees, as well as for the comfort and well-being of their nonsmoking employees. Because of the magnitude of the health effects of smoking and the benefits of cessation, smoking cessation programs are likely to yield a higher return on investment than worksite health promotion programs that target other risk factors such as obesity or lack of exercise. Surveys show that 11% to 15% of American businesses have such antismoking programs, and many more are considering beginning such programs. From one-third to one-half of the large firms in the United States have established no-smoking areas for employees and visitors.

The Health Insurance Association of America has established a program for smoking reduction that is available to its members. Other worksite programs may involve self-help materials, physician messages, and health education lectures, as well as stop-smoking clinics. Stop-smoking sessions have involved coworkers, volunteers from health organizations, commercial consultants, and health professionals. Ongoing multiple risk factor intervention programs, both for smokers and others at risk, may be offered. In order to determine what type of program is best suited for a particular business setting, the advantages and disadvantages of worksite smoking modification programs as contrasted with traditional clinic-based programs are noted in this section. Verification of changes in smoking behavior has become the standard for defining smoking behavior changes; biochemical measures of determining smoking status are noted as being better than reliance on an "informant" who may or may not be able to corroborate smoking behavior objectively.

Worksite Program Effects

The impact of a worksite program may include effects on workers other than those enrolled in a program, and have effects other than smoking cessation. The localized nature of a worksite program and the repetitive interactions of workers in the program with those who did not participate may produce changes in attitudes and behavior of the active workforce that result in the promotion of smoking cessation, and the improvement of employee morale and productivity. For these reasons, a criterion for evaluation of workplace programs should be the fraction of the workforce whose smoking behavior is altered, in addition to the portion of the participants who quit smoking. All these effects are important in evaluating the success rate of a program, because a very high cessation rate for a program may have little overall impact if only small numbers of workers participate. Wherever possible, program costs should be reported in addition to data on the effects of smoking behavior in nonparticipants. Ongoing worksite programs conducted over a period of years should try to document effects of smoking modification programs on variables such as absenteeism, medical care expenses, and health services use.

General Effects

Variables such as employee morale, productivity, commitment to the organization, job turnover, and employee-employer relations are important secondary effects of a worksite anti-smoking program. Because these issues do not directly concern smoking and health, and have been frequently assessed, they are not usually considered. However, it must be noted that the effects of worksite programs must be shown to impact on organizational management goals, because managers may be interested only in managerial results, and not in changes in the health status of employees.

Each component of workplace smoking policies will also create implementation costs. For example, if a smoking policy includes the use of signs to indicate smoking and nonsmoking areas, the costs of the signs will need to be included in any evaluation. While it might be desirable to analyze separately the costs and effects of each component, it is likely to be difficult to access these factors separately.

Even while considering a policy as a whole, it will be difficult to estimate the additional administrative costs that a smoking policy might create for employers. Once they are established and implemented, it is likely that smoking policies will simply be administered along with the other employer policies concerning personnel and buildings. It will thus be difficult to separate the costs of administering the smoking policy from the general costs of administration.

Restrictions on smoking may lead to changes in employee productivity. Some analysts have suggested that smokers are less productive than nonsmokers because of the time lost while smoking. Depending on where smoking is permitted and the design of the workplace, the extent of this possible time loss may change. If smokers need to travel far from their desks to smoke, the total time lost may increase. If they can continue to smoke at their desks, the time lost through smoking will stay the same. If smokers reduce their on-the-job smoking, the amount of time lost may go down. Without the irritation of tobacco smoke, the morale of nonsmokers may improve and they may become more productive. If time has been lost because of conflicts between smokers and nonsmokers concerning where smoking is permitted, implementation of a smoking policy could reduce those conflicts and the consequent productivity loss.

Consideration of Alternatives

An important part of a cost-effectiveness analysis is the consideration of alternatives. Of course, one possible alternative is to do nothing. From a social perspective, no laws or regulations would be enacted. This would leave smokers and nonsmokers, employers and workers, to work out their own arrangements. Under certain very restrictive assumptions concerning the nature of markets and the decisions of employers, workers, and consumers, it has been suggested that a freely operating market system will generate the best possible combination of smoking and nonsmoking policies, prices, and wages. If this is believed to be the case, then there would be no need for additional government action concerning private sector smoking policies. However, the conditions necessary for this conclusion are very restrictive and unlikely to exist.

Beyond the possibility of no action, several alternatives are available to handle the problem of passive smoking; one possibility is to establish smoking policies to designate smoking and nonsmoking areas in the workplace and to make accommodations for the needs of smokers and nonsmokers. Another alternative is physical modification of the workplace to separate smokers' work areas from those of nonsmokers.

Finally, the ventilation system could be redesigned to increase substantially the air flow in all areas to reduce the nonsmokers' exposures to tobacco smoke. For example, the current guidelines of the American Society of Heating, Refrigerating, and Air Conditioning Engineers (ASHRAE) set a ventilation rate of 5 cubic feet per minute of fresh, outside air per person for general offices where smoking is not permitted. For office areas where smoking is permitted, the standard is 20 cubic feet per minute per person. The cost of providing additional ventilation depends on the layout of the building and the amount of heating or cooling that this additional outside air requires. Additional ventilation will also provide an extra benefit by reducing the concentrations of other indoor pollutants to which workers may be exposed. However, stopping smoking is more important in the prevention of respiratory, as well as cardiovascular, disease than is the complete suppression of industrial dust and fumes.[1]

For each of these, a complete listing of the costs and effects would be desirable. However, even without conducting a comprehensive analysis, it appears likely that physical modification of the workplace or the use of additional ventilation would be substantially more expensive than establishing policies concerning smoking in the workplace.

REFERENCE

1. Elmes, P.C. "Relative importance of cigarette smoking in occupational lung disease," *British Journal of Industrial Medicine* 38(1), 1–13, 1981. (NIOSH-00114073)

6

Programs for Smoking Cessation

This chapter discusses the various types of smoking cessation programs available to businesses and individuals, and briefly characterizes each one. Evaluations of programs are briefly provided; the reader is urged to pursue the original literature where the programs are more fully described and discussed.

INCENTIVES FOR QUITTING SMOKING

A number of firms have offered monetary rewards to employees who stop smoking. These incentives range from direct cash payments to bonuses, chances for a raffle, wagers, competitions, and return of fee for attending a cessation clinic. Some firms combine incentives with the hiring of nonsmokers as company policy. The firms that award cash and cash-related bonuses have found that the costs of the awards are less than the cost of the employees' continuing to smoke (in lost time, health problems, and so forth). In a few cases, backsliding employees were required to return a multiple of the bonus (to the American Cancer Society as a donation). Some firms paid part of the employee's cost of a cessation clinic with the stipulation that the firm would reimburse the remainder of the fee if the employee either reduced smoking significantly or quit altogether. Other firms had lotteries, betting on smoking cessation, chances for trips, and raffles, as nonsmoking incentives.

Group penalties were utilized by one firm. Monthly bonuses paid to a participating group of smokers would be forfeited for that month if anyone smoked during working hours; the accumulated bonuses were matched at Christmas by the firm. General success was reported, since group pressure reinforced the nonsmoking edict. Other firms have paid bonuses to workers who quit smoking and remained nonsmoking after attending a nonsmoking clinic; another firm paid team nonsmoking efforts and gave bonuses for group meeting attendance.

The major advantage to incentive programs is that they do not require large amounts of therapist and participant time. These programs are also cost-effective as an approach to smoking on the job, because they cost only when participants are successful in quitting smoking. Biochemical validation is necessary to assure that employees are not "beating the system," because the credibility of the entire incentive program will be severely damaged. The best payoff in terms of getting employees to stop smoking would be to adopt a strict smoking policy, and offer cessation methods combined with incentives to encourage workers to participate in nonsmoking programs and succeed in quitting smoking.

Evaluation of Incentive Programs

In 1977, a small ambulance company began an incentive program for smoking cessation that involved a $5 per month bonus for not smoking at work, for all employees regardless of their initial smoking status. At the end of the year, the owner also matched the total amount of bonuses received during the program. No other intervention techniques were used, and no stop-smoking meetings were held. Another program involved personal incentives, a stop-smoking program, social support, low-calorie food alternatives, and an exercise program. Of 202 employees, 55 enrolled in the program in which each employee who quit smoking for one year received a $200 reward; 31% of the participants reported having successfully stopped smoking for one year. A program involving weekly $7 paycheck bonuses for not smoking at work was studied; after 4 years, only 20% of the employees reported smoking at work compared with 67% before the program began.

A variety of studies have demonstrated that contingent reinforcements for reductions in carbon monoxide levels of expired health samples can produce reliable short-term reductions in carbon monoxide levels in hired smokers. A comprehensive 7-month-long worksite program involving sizable financial incentives as well as health information, social support, and public commitment to nonsmoking in the context of 20 gradually paced group meetings resulted in an 80–91% abstinence rate 6 months after the program began. Unfortunately, most studies that offer incentives for smoking reduction or cessation in the workplace are uncontrolled, and, with notable exceptions, measures of smoking status during nonworking hours and biochemical verification of smoking status are lacking. Incentive programs deserve further investigation, because they are relatively effective, relatively inexpensive, and easy to implement in a variety of settings.

Another approach to providing incentives for improvements in health-related behavior is to arrange competitions among different worksites or teams within a given workplace. Studies of such incentives have reported high participation rates, low attrition rates, and impressive outcome data. In a study of a bank that participated, 88% of all bank employees who were smokers entered the program, compared with another bank in which 53% participated in the same program without competition. However, there were no differences between conditions in cessation rates among participants in the program. The higher participation rate, however, led to a higher long-term cessation rate in the worksite than the comparison condition did.

If the success rate of uncontrolled studies can be replicated in controlled studies, incentive programs may prove to be the most cost-effective approach to workplace smoking modification. However, some people may require additional guidance and support. A convenient, low-cost method of providing skills training in the context of incentive programs is through provision of self-help stop-smoking materials. Although a number of worksite studies have used written self-help materials as part of multicomponent intervention programs, self-help manuals have not been used in incentive programs for smoking cessation, and studies to investigate their unique contribution to treatment outcome have not been conducted.

Overall, the results of incentive- and competition-based programs are very promising. However, almost all of these studies have been conducted in small workplaces, and systematic replications of the findings in controlled studies in larger firms are needed. Nonsmokers should be carefully considered in incentive programs, in their role as supporters of quitters and as nonsmokers, with bonuses for all nonsmokers, old and new, and workplace resources should be provided for all workers.

SMOKING CESSATION PROGRAMS

Numerous firms and public agencies offer direct service health promotion programs to their workers. Areas covered in most of these types of programs include fitness, alcoholism, accident prevention, weight control, stress management, hypertension, nutrition, and smoking. Among the possible mechanisms for accomplishing the sought behavior modification are self-care programs; educational methods, clinics, and groups;

nicotine chewing gum; hypnosis; physician counseling; and behavioral methods. The following smoking cessation methods are offered as possibilities for workplace programs.

EDUCATIONAL PROGRAMS

Educational programs sponsored by companies utilize various methods to bring the antismoking message to employees. Some firms publish articles in company newsletters and bulletins; pamphlets and other educational materials available from health agencies are distributed to employees; posters are displayed in employee lounges and in other areas within the firm; meetings are held where films are shown and talks provided by health professionals. Some firms offer antismoking education during routine health screening examinations. Voluntary health organizations have prepared special promotional materials for workplace use. The American Cancer Society and other organizations provide consultants who assist in designing worksite promotions and help organize orientation meetings.

Self-Care Programs

Self-care means simply being able to perform for oneself activities that maintain health. Self care implies being able to make personal choices based on experience and knowledge; in smoking cessation, self-care consists of devising a personal way of quitting, receiving instructions or advice on how to stop and then doing it, or using aids or self-help guides. Guides for self-care programs often include stop-smoking books or pamphlets, quit kits, instructional manuals, records, cassettes, filters, over-the-counter anti-smoking lozenges, or drug store preparations. In some cases, smokers stop smoking temporarily when they have respiratory disorders involving sore throat, coughing, or colds, or when alarming physical symptoms are experienced, such as loss of breath, chest pains, or weakness. In many cases, smokers do not resume smoking.

Self-care is distinguished from self-management or self-control, because in the latter, behavioral techniques involving other persons (psychologists, for example) are used that negate the self-care aspect. Close management of an individual is not considered self-care. Many cessation methods actually use self-care methods; quitting after a warning from a doctor, or after viewing a television program about quitting, could be termed "self-care"; the impetus for quitting was the warning or the message from the television program.

"Self-help" is often used to mean people helping each other through mutual support groups; this is also part of self-care. Smokers Anonymous encourages smokers to quit and offers support to those who have quit. The National Cancer Institute (NCI) has defined self-help to include an individual or group effort to quit smoking without the continued assistance of professionals, trained leaders, or organizations. This definition included mass media approaches and contact with doctors.

Self-Help Books and Other Self-Help Materials

Numerous self-help books and quit kits are available to guide smokers in their efforts to stop smoking. There are, unfortunately, few evaluations of these materials. The *Self-Testing Kit,* produced by the National Clearinghouse for Smoking and Health in the 1960s, is widely used and is included in most quit books and guides. A *Teenage Self-Test* was also developed by the Clearinghouse. The kits provide an understanding of how one feels about cigarettes, how one uses them, reasons for stopping, and factors that help or hinder the quitting effort. The U.S. Office on Smoking and Health provides smoking cessation pamphlets, such as *Helping Smokers Quit* and *Calling It Quits: The Latest Advice on How to Give Up Cigarettes*. NCI designed the *Helping Smokers Quit Kit* which contains materials for the smoker and the physician. The *Quit for Good Kit* replaced the earlier kit, and is designed for doctors and dental and other health professionals to use in counseling patients. The kit contains two patient brochures, *Quit It* and *For*

Good, with cessation and maintenance tips. NCI recently developed a *Helping Smokers Quit Kit* for pharmacists to use in counseling people on quitting. NCI also offers *Clearing the Air,* which details methods and techniques for smoking cessation. A Spanish version is available. NCI makes available a supplemental factsheet, *You've Kicked the Smoking Habit—For Good!* that provides a variety of tips for maintenance.

In 1977, the American Cancer Society (ACS) developed the *I Quit Kit* that contains portions of the 1960 *Self-Test,* instructions for quitting over a 7-day period, a quitting calendar, a phonograph record that details experiences in quitting, breathing exercises, songs, skits, a poster, tips on quitting and remaining off smoking, and I Quit buttons. The *Quit Kit,* developed by Stanford University, consists of an explanatory flier, sheets with behavioral tips for quitting smoking, and a 2-inch heart magnet.

The American Lung Association (ALA) produced two manuals for people wishing to quit on their own: *Freedom From Smoking in 20 Days,* a 64-page guide, and a 28-page maintenance guide, *A Lifetime of Freedom From Smoking.* The cessation guide includes part of the 1960 *Self-Test,* a cigarette record, contracts to sign, and describes triggers to smoking. Weight control techniques, methods for handling smoking situations, and deep-breathing and muscle relaxation techniques are offered. Tasks and information are offered for each of 20 days, with the first 7 days considered as preparation, the next 9 days quitting, and the last 4 days reinforcement of nonsmoking behavior. The maintenance booklet supports the ex-smoker by providing techniques for coping with smoking urges; diet information, tension relief techniques, and social situations are treated. A recently produced (1989) program designed for corporate settings is the LIFESIGN program, a self-contained, self-administered program tailored to the user's individual smoking habit and lifestyle.

There are numerous "quit smoking" books on the market; a few are summarized here. *Break the Cigarette Habit—A Behavioral Program for Giving Up Cigarettes* depends on behavioral modification techniques, leading the smoker through gradual reduction to complete abstinence. Stimulus control techniques are presented, and weight gain and other problems arising from quitting are discussed. *Stop Smoking for Good* and *No More Butts—A Psychologist's Approach to Quitting Cigarettes* also utilize behavior modification techniques. *You Can Stop: A SmokEnder Approach to Quitting Smoking and Sticking to It* emphasizes careful preparation and development of the proper attitude for quitting. Case histories, relaxation, diet, and exercise suggestions are included. *The Joy of Quitting* is directed at teenagers; it summarizes the effects of smoking and excuses for not stopping are discussed. Diet and quitting methods are presented. *Quit Smoking in 30 Days* includes preparation, quitting, and maintenance phases; tips are provided on how to deal with withdrawal symptoms, weight gain, and potential relapse. *Quit Smoking* discusses the psychology and physiology of cigarette use and describes ways of quitting. *The Smoker's Book of Health: How to Keep Yourself Healthier and Cut Your Smoking Risk* advises smokers on how to improve their health and offers methods and tips to those contemplating quitting. Eating, exercise, stress reduction, and social support are discussed. *The Stop Smoking Diet,* a diet book, assumes nicotine to be the addictive component of cigarettes. Diets designed to eliminate nicotine from the body are given, and a diet change is presented for use when smoking is stopped. (Unfortunately, the author also offers smoking substitutes which may be unhealthy.)

Audiovisual materials are also available to help the potential quitter: *In Control,* a 2-hour video program produced by the ALA, is available to those who have VCRs at home. A viewer's guide, audiocassette with motivational and relaxational messages, and a 14-day weight maintenance program are also included. Recently available are 60-minute audiotapes that carry positive affirmations and relaxation techniques to help people gain the will power to stop smoking; two different tapes are available, one for women, and the other for men.

Aids to Quitting

A variety of aids are available to help the smoker quit; however, their effectiveness is questionable. The most popular aid is a filter that reduces tar, nicotine, and carbon monoxide levels, permitting the smoker to be weaned from the chemical addiction of smoking. Over-the-counter products that are taken internally as aids to smoking cessation are available; Bantron is a well-known brand. Chewing gums and lozenges are also available, as is a "smokeless cigarette"; other products include tobacco-less "cigarettes" that smell like tobacco but do not contain nicotine. The Food and Drug Administration (FDA) is currently investigating such deterrents; unfortunately, some of the ingredients in the products tested are neither safe or effective. A discussion of several types of pharmacological products used in quitting smoking are presented in a National Institute on Drug Abuse monograph.[1]

Quitting by Mail

Studies have been made on the effectiveness of quitting by mail, which involves sending materials to those unable or unwilling to attend therapy in person. This type of approach blends self-help and therapy sessions, and allows people to quit on their own, while providing the support of a group session. Computerized programs are also available; however, these are intended for distribution by firms to their employees.

EDUCATIONAL METHODS, CLINICS, AND GROUPS

Various techniques are available to employers who wish to use programs developed by public and private agencies; these programs are sponsored by a variety of organizations such as schools, colleges, medical centers, religious groups, research foundations, medical societies, interagency councils, military units, rural community and service agencies, labor unions, and exercise clubs, as well as private businesses at offices and factories. Many of these programs are based on programs or materials supplied by non-profit groups such as ALA or ACS and religious groups such as the Seventh-Day Adventist Church, but many clinics offer biofeedback, hypnosis, behavioral approaches, or their own methods. Smokeless and SmokeStoppers are popular programs in hospitals.

Educational Methods Available From Nonprofit and Public Agencies

The annual report of the Surgeon General, prepared by the Office on Smoking and Health (OSH) (*The Health Consequences of Smoking*), together with announcements and publications from other government and voluntary agencies, provide the public and the employer with incentives and ways to quit smoking. The OSH offers educational materials, bibliographies, and scientific findings related to smoking and stopping smoking. The 1960 *Self Test Kit* was mentioned in a previous section. OSH publishes the annual report on the health consequences of smoking and conducts surveys of smoking habits and attitudes among adults, teenagers, and health professionals. OSH published the ongoing *Bibliography on Smoking and Health,* which summarizes the world literature on smoking and health. This is an important information resource for the scientific community about prevention and withdrawal methods.

Several other governmental agencies, the National Cancer Institute; National Heart, Lung, and Blood Institute; Centers for Disease Control; National Institute of Child Health and Human Development; and the National Institute on Drug Abuse publish materials on smoking cessation and fund research, and sponsor conferences on smoking prevention and cessation.

In Canada, the Ministry of National Health and Welfare directs a national effort to reduce cigarette smoking, including the production of educational materials, films, and TV clips; coordinating professional activities; funding research programs; and conducting national surveys of smoking attitudes and habits. In 1982, the Ministry, in collaboration with provincial health departments and major voluntary health associations, initiated a major smoking prevention program, Towards a Generation of Nonsmokers, or briefly, "Generation." The program aims to create an awareness of the consequences of smoking, encourage cessation, and foster a nonsmoking social environment. The Time to Quit program focuses on current smokers, and uses a multimedia, community-based approach.

The American Cancer Association (ACS) is prominent in smoking prevention and cessation programming. In addition to publishing educational materials and quit guides, the Association has produced cessation trigger films, funded cessation studies, participated in public policy programs, sponsored scientific and lay conferences on smoking cessation, and provided professional education on smoking control to health care professionals. In addition to numerous international and national conferences, the ACS began the Great American Smokeout as an annual cessation event that continues to be noticed by the media.

ACS has active withdrawal programs for adults and teenagers and sponsors a smoker's telephone quit-line. ACS, recognizing the limitations of local ACS groups, has been placing priority attention on preparing representatives of business and industry, schools, hospitals, clubs, and other organizations to conduct cessation programs on their own. The Association's *Quitter's Guide* and *I Quit Kit* are made available to local units who are encouraged to install recorded telephone messages and locate volunteer ex-smokers to help current smokers with quitting. FreshStart is a program that compresses the former 16-hour program into 4 hours; local ACS units train representatives to become FreshStart facilitators.

The American Lung Association, in line with its goal of cleaning up the air, discourages smoking through public policy activities, public education programs, workshops for professionals, and funding research and community activities. Local associations give help to smokers wishing to quit by offering materials, consultation, and cessation clinics.

In 1975, ALA, the American Thoracic Society, and the Congress of Lung Association Staff together launched a project to develop stop-smoking programs that used self-help, clinic, and mass media approaches. The project produced two manuals in workbook format, *Freedom From Smoking in 20 Days* and *A Lifetime of Freedom From Smoking*. The former manual is a systematic day-by-day approach leading to complete cessation on the 16th day with 4 follow-up days to cope with the initial difficulties of quitting. The latter manual is designed to be used by the ex-smoker to maintain nonsmoking. The manuals are also used in a clinic format with the leader offering encouragement and the group providing support. ALA has adapted the manual for workplace use, and ALA staff help firms to develop quitting programs.

The Canadian Council on Smoking and Health, formed in 1974, fosters interagency cooperation with a priority to form provincial and local councils on smoking and health. The Council cooperates with the national government in promoting the Generation program. The Council sponsors an annual National Non-Smoking Week during January. Weedless Wednesday is a national nonsmoking day that encourages the one-day-at-a-time approach to quitting smoking; public and private health organizations cooperate to make Weedless Wednesday a media event. The Council also sponsors conferences and workshops on smoking cessation.

The Canadian Cancer Society and the Canadian federal government developed the Time to Quit program, a cognitive-behavioral approach based on the health belief model (belief in personal susceptibility). The smoker examines problems connected with quitting and practices strategies for coping with these problems. The program consists of 3 half-hour television programs, self-help booklets, and a community guide.

The Canadian Heart Foundation and the Canadian Lung Association promote a variety of programs to build the public's awareness of nonsmoking benefits. Local units have sponsored cessation programs, notably Countdown, a 7-session, 5-week tapering-off cessation course consisting of both self-help and clinic portions.

Educational Techniques

It is difficult to classify smoking cessation methods into categories; educational and group methods have many techniques in common. Any method that assembles people into some type of group might result in group support; almost all programs have educational components when they provide facts about the harmful effects of smoking and the benefits of nonsmoking.

In addition to prevention programs, many schools sponsor cessation classes for high school students and adults. Some states use the ACS clinic format, others use decision making, self-management skills, and group support activities. Some schools confer credits on students for smoking cessation classes. Colleges and universities also offer withdrawal methods, some use the ACS FreshStart method, others use hypnosis and relaxation techniques.

Educational cessation methods generally consist of lectures by health professionals, films, records of smoking, literature, quitting instructions, diet information, and answers to questions. Frequently, the "buddy" system is used for support. Treatment sessions may last from one week to three months. Usually the approach is didactic, and conversation is between the leader and a participant. Some programs are held in hospitals, and doctors function as leaders; chronic obstructive pulmonary disease can then be emphasized as a consequence of smoking. In some programs, groups visit the pulmonary disease intensive care unit.

Some industry clinics are educational; lectures, films, counseling, and the "buddy" system are used. Stop-smoking materials are also distributed, and abstinence verification techniques are used. Other groups, notably religious groups, and especially the Seventh-Day Adventist Church, have developed very useful programs. The Adventist Five-Day Plan has been widely copied and adapted by professionals and laypersons; over 14 million smokers have entered the program in over 150 countries. It has been offered in settings ranging from prisons to commuter trains, and is available via films.

The Five-Day Plan charges a small fee for materials costs, and consists of five consecutive 90-minute or 2-hour sessions, with several weekly follow-up meetings. At the first meeting, a film showing surgery on a cancerous lung is usually shown. Cessation is immediate, and coffee, tea, cola, and alcohol are also temporarily prohibited. Physical fitness, exercise, a balanced diet, whole grain breads and cereals, avoidance of saturated fats and highly-spiced foods, vitamins, forced intake of fluids, warm baths, hot and cold showers, body rubs, deep breathing, prayer, and a "buddy" system are encouraged. Sessions discuss the physiological effects of smoking, and actual lung specimens are displayed. Clergymen, psychologists, and doctors present spiritual, mental, or medical lectures and conduct counseling sessions. One or two maintenance sessions are usually held, with very high quit rates reported, especially when assessments are on the last night of the program. The Plan has been used by some firms in occupational settings, with moderate success reported. (The Adventist church now has changed the name for copyright purposes and for the exclusive use of the church. Some other changes have also been made.)

The Plan now features motivation and lifestyle modification strategies in additional to self-rewards; other rewards include the I Love Being Free From Smoking! button for 24 hours of nonsmoking; a diploma on graduation called B.N.S. (Bachelor of Nonsmoking); a silver seal added to the diploma for attending every session; a gold seal for nonsmoking after the third session; an M.N.S. diploma (Master of Nonsmoking) after 6 months, and lastly, a D.N.S. diploma (Doctorate of Nonsmoking) 12 months after graduating. The new 8-week length of the program is divided over 3 weeks; two sessions the first week held 48 hours apart, five consecutive sessions the second week, and a final graduation session the third week. Quitting will be by the third session, and encouraging telephone calls are made 1 week and 3, 6, and 12 months after graduation. Each session includes lectures, discussions, a film, and take-home material. The Plan is nondenominational and has a strong but optional spiritual emphasis.

Another type of educational program that uses the Five-Day Plan is an in-residence treatment; the Plan uses a live-in setting with exercise therapists, dietitians, physical therapists, health educators, nurses, and doctors. Fees range from $995 to $1195 and cover group sessions, lectures, films, private rooms with baths, 5 days of meals, use of pool and sauna, a pulmonary function study, consultation with a physician, and weight, tension, physical conditioning, and physical therapy sessions. Participants have daily calisthenics, relaxation exercises, steam baths, lectures, and films. Vegetarian food is served, and coffee, tea, colas, and alcohol are prohibited. Liberal intake of fruit juices and water are encouraged. Follow-up studies have indicated that after 1 year, 30% of participants were abstinent. Motivation is high among participants because of the financial investment, time investment, and travel expenses. Attendees receive newsletters and a toll-free telephone number is provided for consultation with staff.

Withdrawal Clinics and Groups

Most withdrawal clinics use the group approach, but there may be large differences between a group led by a trained leader and one led by a volunteer ex-smoker with no previous group training. There may also be differences between a therapy group that runs 5 consecutive days and one that lasts 6 to 8 weeks. It takes several weeks for group members to get acquainted, become comfortable in admitting difficulties in quitting, and offer support to each other.

The ACS conducts smoking cessation clinics through its divisions and local units. The program has been widely used in the community, industry, hospitals, the military, and schools. The Helping Smokers Quit clinics are a mix of educational and group approach; it is standardized throughout the United States, via the use of guides, printed materials, and trigger films presented by trained volunteers. Interaction of the 15 to 20 group members promotes personal growth and later reinforces abstinence. A specific session-by-session format is required, though it may be modified somewhat to take advantage of the leader's capabilities and the relative sophistication of the clinic participants.

The clinic has three phases: self-appraisal and insight development; practicing abstinence under controlled conditions; and a maintenance phase that varies according to the wishes of each participant. Groups meet for eight 2-hour sessions, usually twice weekly. One trigger film lasting for 3–8 minutes is shown at each session; the films are designed to stimulate discussion and help smokers react to the quitting process. Buddies are chosen during the first phase for ongoing support, and participants are encouraged to form an IQ (I Quit) Club to reinforce continued nonsmoking. There is little followup maintenance after smokers have finished the program; a $25 contribution is requested but not mandatory.

A shorter and more concentrated version of the ACS clinic also was effective; surveys have shown that marathon sessions were less effective and more difficult to conduct. Based on these changes, ACS developed the new quit-smoking program, FreshStart, which consisted of four 1-hour, small group sessions. Reading assignments follow each meeting to help participants keep in mind what has been discussed. The first session provides an understanding of why people smoke and the effects of smoking. Approaches to quitting are outlined with "cold turkey" recommended. The second session deals with withdrawal symptoms; four counteractive behaviors are suggested. Practicing stress management and assertiveness are other suggested activities. The third session handles obstacles such as weight gain. The fourth session includes tips to help the person stay off cigarettes. Those persons failing to quit are encouraged to rejoin a new group or to quit on their own. Graduates of the FreshStart program are recruited to serve as group leaders or responders on the Smoker's Quitline.

The American Lung Association (ALA) emphasizes self-help and media approaches, but also sponsors a clinic program. Some individual chapters have formulated their own methods; the Washington Lung Association's Kick the Idiotic Cigarette Habit consists of a 6-session program with participants going "cold turkey" in the first session. UNsmoke is an 8-week group class sponsored by the Lung Association of Hennepin County, Minnesota. Some 50 visual aids are used during the classes, and nonsmoking status is validated at followup sessions by chemical means.

The Tuberculosis-Christmas Seal Society of British Columbia sponsored KICK-IT, and the Manitoba Lung Association conducts Operation Kick-It with 8 weekly meetings with a trained volunteer ex-smoker leader. The ALA of Southeastern

Michigan developed a 3-hour withdrawal clinic, Cigarette Send-Off, which uses hypnotherapy as well as cognitive and behavioral techniques. Chronic respiratory patients and doctors give presentations, and films are shown. Public vows to quit and the throwing away of cigarettes end the session.

The American Health Foundation (AHF) has run an active cessation program for many years; the methods used include self-help, individual counseling, self-hypnosis, and groups. AHF works with corporations to advise them on cessation activities and to train company personnel to conduct programs.

PHYSICIAN-MEDIATED STOP SMOKING PROGRAMS

Physician Counseling

Because as many as 70% of adults in our country visit their doctor at least yearly, there has been interest in finding ways in which doctors can convince patients to give up smoking. National surveys have indicated that a high proportion of doctors believe that it is their responsibility to help their patients to stop smoking and that they should convince people to quit. However, physicians are reluctant to counsel their patients to quit smoking until serious health problems are present. Physicians had little confidence in their ability to help patients to change smoking behavior, even though they were better prepared to offer counseling about smoking than about other behaviors. Most smokers state that they are aware of the health risks of smoking, and they view the physician as an important person in their decision to quit smoking. The proportion of doctors that smoke has declined to about 10%, and there are indications that more doctors are advising and counseling their patients about stopping smoking.

Studies done in Europe have found that a greater number of individuals at high risk for developing heart disease stopped smoking when a doctor advised them, at least semi-annually, than did individuals in a control group. However, some studies showed that there was no difference in the quitting rates of groups exposed to physician messages as compared to control groups that did not have physician advice. There are both advantages and disadvantages to using physician stop-smoking messages in workplace settings; one advantage is that if stop-smoking advice is incorporated into regularly scheduled physician visits, a relatively large number of workers can be advised and treated quickly and effectively. Another advantage of the physician advice treatment is that it is relatively unobtrusive in comparison with management-sponsored programs. Physician advice can be used to augment other intervention methods without replacing them, by assisting workers in deciding to seek help and by promoting participation in intervention programs, therefore making better use of these programs. A monograph with suggested programs for doctor-assisted intervention is listed in the bibliography at the end of this chapter.[2]

Although self-reported cessation rates resulting from physician advice are low, research is underway to attempt to increase the impact of stop-smoking messages. Research has found that implementation of a 3- to 5-minute session of behavioral counseling by staff physicians at a navy shipyard clinic significantly increased stop-smoking rates over those resulting from a simple warning to quit smoking. In addition, the compliance of health care providers with treatment protocols also affects outcome. For example, researchers reported that it was difficult to get doctors to deliver a brief message to patients, but provision of feedback to doctors appears to improve quality and quantity of stop-smoking messages. Perhaps a stop-smoking message together with other intervention techniques might increase success rates.

Basic research on the effects of threatening messages such as those describing health risks of smoking indicates that such messages have their greatest impact if individuals know not only what to do but how to do it, and believe themselves capable of acting. The approval of nicotine chewing gum and the availability of high quality self-help stop-smoking manuals present opportunities for doctors to deliver health warnings together with concrete recommendations for what to do and how to do it. Recent data suggest that nicotine chewing gum may help heavy smokers to quit, and gum prescriptions can be written at the same time that a stop-smoking message is given.

Medication

Medication as an adjunct to smoking cessation has been in existence since the early 1900s. Lobeline sulfate, one of the earliest materials used, has unpleasant side effects that now have been minimized by using antacids together with the lobeline products. Tablets and lozenges containing this material are sold over-the-counter and dispensed to attendees at many stop-smoking clinics. Over the last few years, lobeline products have largely been replaced by nicotine chewing gum. One such product is Bantron, an over-the-counter material; others are Health-break and Ban Smoke, which contain other materials. The Public Citizen Health Research Group, in a series of articles on stopping smoking, has indicated that these materials are ineffective.

Numerous other drugs are available to counter withdrawal symptoms of smoking cessation; these include meprobamate, d-amphetamine, methylscopolamine, mecamylamine, propanolol, clonidine, aprazolam, and drugs that are categorized as anticholinerics, sedatives, sympathomimetics, and anticonvulsants. Placebos have also been used effectively in smoking cessation. The drugs work in several different ways to offer some relief to smoking cessation problems; however, none appear to be ideal and they may present more risks than benefits.

Nicotine Chewing Gum

The most effective substance to date that has been used in smoking cessation programs is nicotine chewing gum. Researchers believe that it is effective because it contains the same habit-forming material as do cigarettes. It is sold in the United States by prescription as Nicorette; it is available in some countries as an over-the-counter material. Cardiovascular studies have shown that smoking a cigarette or chewing Nicorette causes very similar physiological effects. The differences were a more rapid increase in heart rate and blood pressure after smoking but a more prolonged elevation of these parameters after chewing Nicorette containing 4 mg of nicotine. The 2 mg dose of Nicorette was similar to a cigarette in terms of the time course of the response. The only dosage approved by the Food and Drug Administration in the United States is the 2 mg Nicorette. The majority of smokers are satisfied with 2 mg Nicorette, even though blood nicotine levels are lower than when smoking cigarettes, because the lower nicotine blood level is enough to alleviate withdrawal symptoms in the serious quitter.

Side effects of Nicorette are related to nicotine and to gum chewing. Nicotine effects may be local (oral irritation) or systemic; gum chewing may produce local (dental trauma), mechanical (jaw muscle ache), or gastrointestinal effects. Adverse effects reported for Nicorette include excess salivation, insomnia, dizziness, irritability, headache, nonspecific gastrointestinal distress, belching, indigestion, nausea, vomiting, mouth or throat soreness, jaw muscle ache, anorexia, and hiccups. Patients are encouraged to chew the gum slowly to release the nicotine gradually, and to minimize side effects.

Nicorette is contraindicated in patients who have recently suffered myocardial infarction, patients with life-threatening arrhythmias, patients with severe or worsening angina pectoris, and patients with active temporomandibular joint disease. Nicorette should not be used by pregnant or nursing women, and caution should be taken by patients with oral or pharyngeal inflammation or with a history of esophagitis or peptic ulcer.

Nicorette is a prescription drug in the form of sugar-free chewing gum containing nicotine bound to an ion-exchange resin that allows for slow release of nicotine during chewing. The gum is buffered to allow absorption of nicotine in the mouth. The manufacturer, Merrell Dow, makes available a *Physician's Quitting Source Kit for Nicorette* and *Instructions for Use*. The patient starting on Nicorette is asked to stop smoking and chew a piece of gum slowly whenever he or she feels the need to smoke. The instructions advise against chewing more than 30 pieces of gum per day. The patient is advised to gradually reduce the number of pieces of gum chewed per day as the urge to smoke fades. The instructions advise the patient not to stop using the gum until one or two pieces of gum a day satisfies the craving. The patient is advised not to use the gum for more than 6 months. Costs of a 3-month supply of Nicorette gum is about $225.00, plus doctor's fees and any costs for a supplementary program or self-help materials.

Researchers have advised that Nicorette be used as part of a general stop-smoking program rather than by itself; it should be regarded as an aid to smoking cessation and not as a long-term tobacco substitute. Evaluation of stop-smoking programs using Nicorette has shown that nicotine chewing gum can be an effective tool in achieving abstinence from cigarettes if some type of support, counseling, or therapy is provided. Doctors are advised to proceed with caution in prescribing nicotine gum; the gum should not be used indiscriminately in lieu of an adequate support system. The gum has potential addictive properties; patients often have unrealistic expectations of the gum; patients may not, despite package instructions, chew properly, resulting in the production of undesirable side effects. Patients must realize that nicotine from gum is absorbed much more slowly and that the gum will not duplicate the effects of cigarettes.

The Public Citizen Health Research Group has suggested the Nicorette system together with physician counseling as the best method for quitting smoking. The Group cautions that the gum is habit-forming, and for some smokers who are heavily addicted to nicotine, the gum may replace smoking. Thus it is very important to have a physician well-versed in smoking cessation and the concomitant addiction problems to administer this type of program. Nicotine gum has been found to enhance treatment outcome in self-help conditions, but during some types of programs, subjects receiving the gum had lower cessation rates than did subjects not receiving the gum.

Hypnosis

Hypnosis has become very popular as a smoking cessation method, but there are contradictory reports of its effectiveness. Numerous accounts describe the use of hypnosis with small numbers of patients, but only a limited number of reports are based on follow-up data or state whether patients actually quit smoking. Some hypnotists claim good results based on estimates or faulty evaluations. One critique states that hypnosis, although not a potent means of controlling behavior, is uniquely effective in helping individuals to do what they want to do. The patient must assume responsibility for changing his own behavior and must recognize that failure can only be blamed on himself or herself, not on the therapist. Hypnosis is usually presented together with some form of behavior therapy, and is not the sole form of intervention in smoking. According to an article published by the Public Citizen Health Research Group and based on reviews of over 50 studies, hypnosis is an interventional method that does not work. The group cited a lack of controlled studies needed to validate claims.

Acupuncture

Acupuncture is based on the Chinese science of connections in the body. Use is made of needles or staple-like attachments to treat the smoker. The method is painful. The method has gained in popularity since the late 1970s, when it was first introduced as a stop-smoking method. As in the case of hypnosis, studies are inconclusive as to efficacy in helping smokers to quit; followup studies are incomplete and evaluative studies were ill-designed. Some researchers claim that acupuncture works because of the placebo effect; the needles do nothing, but the patient thinks that they do, and is helped to quit smoking. The Public Citizen Health Research Group has labeled this method as ineffective due to lack of evaluative research. Acupuncture is also costly, with doctors charging up to $60 a session.

BEHAVIORAL METHODS FOR STOPPING SMOKING

Behavioral modifiction methods for smoking cessation belong to two major categories: aversive procedures, and self-management procedures. Aversive methods are further divided into rapid smoking, other smoke aversion procedures, covert sensitization, and shock therapy. Self-management methods are subdivided into self-monitoring, nicotine fading, stimulus control, contingency management, systematic desensitization and relaxation, sensory deprivation, and self-control procedures.

Aversive Procedures

Aversive agents or techniques include electric shock, breath holding, smoke, unpleasant taste, noise, or smell, and imagined stimuli. The principles of extinction, negative practice, and aversive conditioning employ stimuli from cigarettes themselves as the aversive component, such as rapid smoking and satiation smoking. These procedures are based on two assumptions: first, that the reinforcing aspects of almost any stimulus are reduced and may actually become aversive if that stimulus is presented at sufficiently elevated frequency or intensity; and second, that aversion based upon stimuli intrinsic to the target response (smoking) is more salient and generalized than that stemming from artificial sources.

Past reviews of smoking modification research indicate that aversive techniques largely have failed to help people to quit smoking. The most promising techniques use some form of smoke aversion.

Rapid Smoking

Blowing warm, stale smoke in subjects' faces while they smoked was introduced in 1964, but showed only limited success. The procedure was modified by several researchers, and the combination of rapid smoking with self-control and counseling has had the best results for this type of aversion procedure. There has been concern about the effects of rapid smoking on the cardiopulmonary system; increased amounts of nicotine could induce cardiac arrhythmias in people with coronary artery disease. Rapid smoking produces clinically significant hypoxemia (insufficient blood oxygenation) in some persons. Increases in heart rate, blood pressure, and carboxyhemoglobin levels as well as electrocardiographic abnormalities have been noted in some subjects undergoing rapid smoking aversion programs. However, according to some researchers, rapid smoking aversion techniques are safe for healthy young adults.

Rapid smoking techniques appear to produce high quit rates at the end of treatment; inclusion of other procedures, such as self-control, physical examinations, and relapse training, improve the quit rate dramatically.

Factors necessary for rapid smoking to succeed in producing long-term success are as follows. A warm, supportive therapist is required to supervise therapy, and the therapist must heighten the subject's awareness of the aversion and admonish the subject not to smoke between sessions. The process of revivification should be used to enhance the aversion between rapid smoking sessions. Treatment should continue until the subject experiences no more urges to smoke, usually after 7 or 8 sessions.

In view of the acute effects that rapid smoking has on the cardiopulmonary system, care should be taken to screen subjects and monitor them closely during treatment. Persons with cardiac disease should be treated with rapid smoking only if medical backup is available.

Other Smoke Aversion Procedures

In addition to rapid smoking, other smoke aversion methods are the use of smoky air, smoke satiation, chain smoking, regular paced aversive smoking, and smoke holding. Blowing warm, stale smoke in the subject's face was noted in previous sections. This procedure involves the use of a cumbersome apparatus, and no studies reported the use of this procedure after 1977.

Satiation subjects are required to increase the number of cigarettes smoked, not the rate at which they are smoked. The amount of smoking and duration varies according to the experiment; usually the subject is required to double or triple the baseline amount smoked. Satiation is generally done at home, which creates monitoring and compliance problems. Satiation requires no apparatus but does require health screening of subjects because satiation produces high doses of nicotine that could aversely affect the cardiopulmonary system.

Satiation is most successful when combined with other procedures, including smoky air, rapid smoking, self-control, desensitization, contractual management, group support, and special maintenance procedures. However, satiation is not considered as effective as rapid smoking techniques.

Another form of oversmoking, chain smoking, has had some success, as has regular paced aversive smoking; this type of procedure, called focused smoking, is used to avoid the risks posed by rapid smoking and satiation. It is delivered in a variety of ways; generally, subjects smoke at their usual rate while focusing on the negative features of cigarettes, such as mouth and throat irritation, coughing, and the accumulation of smoke. Some researchers have had subjects view lists of antismoking statements while they were in the regular paced smoking program; other subjects have had to listen to a therapist point out the aversive aspects of cigarettes while they puffed every 30 seconds. Focused smoking is a more successful quitting method if it is combined with physiological measures. Regular paced smoking has an advantage over rapid smoking in that it does not require extra health screening.

Taste satiation or smoke holding until discomfort occurs appears to be a safe procedure and has the advantage of not requiring special screening procedures. Unfortunately, not enough data are available to permit assessment of the efficacy of smoke holding by itself as a cessation treatment.

Covert Sensitization

The objective of covert sensitization is to produce avoidance behavior through the use of the subject's imagination. Both the behavior to be modified and the noxious stimulus are imagined. Researchers believe that this procedure is analogous to a punishment routine because the smoker is asked to imagine that he or she is receiving noxious stimulation while associating cigarettes with aversive thoughts. The subject can also imagine positive consequences when thinking of not smoking. It appears that covert sensitization together with other treatment procedures have been more effective than the procedure by itself.

Covert sensitization combined with relaxation techniques have been successful, because there is a need to deal with tension surrounding the need to smoke. Rapid smoking procedures combined with covert sensitization have also been somewhat successful in producing quitting.

Shock Therapy

The use of electric shock as a punishing stimulus to eliminate smoking behavior has been used with limited success. No reports of smoking cessation trials using this technique were noted after 1977. Some techniques do not use electric shock but utilize a rubber band worn around one wrist; the subject is instructed to snap the band when thoughts leading to smoking were present. Alternate behaviors, such as gum chewing, were suggested to replace the smoking thoughts at that time. For some subjects, wearing the rubber band as a reminder was successful. Women were not as successful with this technique as men. The procedure, although painful, does not appear to arouse as much anxiety as electric shock does.

Self-Management Techniques

Strategies for quitting smoking through self-management include a number of techniques, some of which are used with aversive methods. Self-control programs are not self-initiated, but they include both self-administered programs and those involving a leader or therapist. (The reader is reminded of the difference between self-care and self-mangement or self-control methods.) The latter are behavioral techniques, generally initated and directed by leaders and therapists, that usually include supervision.

The use of self-control evolves from three factors: first, attention to one's own smoking actions and recording their occurrences; second, the awareness of and willingness to change one's environment so that either the cues preceding the smoking response or the immediate consequences of it are changed; and third, recognition of and ability to break long-standing, cue-elicited smoking patterns. The usual self-control program involves the subject more actively in treatment than do aversive methods.

Predominant self-management methods are those based on concepts of self-monitoring, nicotine fading, stimulus control, contingency management, systematic desensitization and relaxation, restricted environmental stimulation therapy, and self-control packages.

Self-Monitoring

Keeping records of the number of cigarettes smoked has been required by almost all smoking cessation programs to assess baseline smoking, progress in treatment, and outcome. Program requirements regarding self-monitoring have differed from counting cigarettes smoked for just one day to elaborately recording for one week the time, place, activity, and mood when smoking each cigarette and the need for it.

Studies have shown that focusing on positive instances of smoking (rewards) increases the frequency of smoking while decreasing the time spent per cigarette and that focusing on negative consequences of smoking decreases smoking frequency while also decreasing time per cigarette. Smoking duration and frequency are also affected by self-monitoring, which indicates that it is a reactive data-gathering procedure (producing its own behavior changes). One researcher has stated that self-monitoring can be useful provided that self-monitoring assignments are not overly complex, are varied or are not continuously required throughout a lengthy program, and are not focused solely on "negative" targets such as withdrawal symptoms. As in other self-directed programs, the need to validate self-reports by physiological measurements is present in the self-monitoring program area also.

Nicotine Fading

Cutting down on the number of cigarettes smoked based on weekly goals has been used as a cessation method for many years. Generally called gradual withdrawal or tapering, this method was advocated for "habit" smokers in contrast to cold turkey, which was advocated for "negative effect" smokers. Smoke Watchers bases its program on gradual withdrawal and weekly goals assigned by the group leader; clients are praised by the group when they meet their goals. The rationale for nicotine fading differs from that of gradual reduction in numbers of cigarettes. Although Smoke Watchers has had some success with tapering, the evidence for gradual reduction in numbers is not very positive. As cigarettes are reduced, each remaining cigarette can become more reinforcing. With nicotine fading, however, individuals can continue to smoke the same number of cigarettes. By recording nicotine content over several brand changes, participants can perceive considerable progress in nicotine reduction (even though much of this decrease is illusory).

Nicotine or brand fading by changing one's brand of cigarettes is a relatively new treatment method, introduced in 1978. Brands are switched in the direction of gradually lowering the nicotine intake to wean the smoker from his or her nicotine dependence. The nicotine content of cigarettes is derived from figures published by the Federal Trade Commission. Some treatment procedures have combined nicotine fading with other behavioral modification procedures, with moderate success. Physiological monitoring methods must be utilized to assure than the subjects have indeed switched to lower-nicotine brands, and are not smoking more on their own, to make up for the lack of nicotine. Considered together with other behavioral methods, nicotine fading has good possibilities for successful application in a smoking cessation program.

Stimulus Control

As a clinical procedure, stimulus control seeks to eliminate undesirable behaviors by altering the prevailing stimulus situations in which the maladaptive response occurs. Smoking is generally associated with a variety of specific environmental and internal events. These associations trigger the smoking response. Certain associations reinforce that response. The prevailing stimulus-response conditions are generally altered via a two-step stimulus control program consisting of the following: (1) smoking is initially restricted to novel situations in order to extinguish the power of prior cues, and (2) the novel stimuli are subsequently faded, thereby encouraging a corresponding reduction/elimination of smoking. Stimulus control treatments emphasize gradual reduction instead of immediate cessation and can take a variety of forms.

Various investigators list three strategies for achieving stimulus control of smoking. The first, increasing the stimulus interval, allows continued smoking but limits smoking to particular times that are signaled by some cuing device, for instance, a pocket timer. Once well established, the new smoking cue is gradually faded out simply by increasing the time interval. The second strategy is hierarchical reduction. Subjects are asked to monitor their smoking activity carefully and to identify situations in which smoking would have a high or low probability of occurring. A hierarchy is developed based either on the presumed difficulty of reducing smoking in a situation or on the enjoyment derived from smoking in the situation. The subject then reduces or eliminates smoking in cumulative and progressive fashion from the easiest to the hardest situation in the hierarchy. The third strategy is deprived response performance. This method progressively narrows the discriminative stimuli for smoking by limiting the circumstances in which smoking is allowed. The procedure requires that all smoking occur in a deprived setting, one devoid of all possible distractions and accompanying reinforcers.

The predominant technique under the first classification is using a signal or timer device that interferes with the normal smoking responses. Some studies have had the subjects smoke on a new cue presented at random times by a portable signaling device. The substitute cue is initially set at the smoker's normal rate and then gradually phased out. Such a study, primarily designed to test the feasibility of the method, indicated that people who followed the program reduced their smoking more than those who dropped out of the program.

The second classification of stimulus control is hierarchical reduction. Studies have found that having a target quitting date was significantly more effective than gradual quitting. Delaying the quit date was more effective than quitting immediately for women but less so for men. Some researchers have found that having subjects keep detailed records of each cigarette smoked (time, feelings, and need) was helpful, because smoking is a learned behavior in response to internal signals (thoughts and emotions) and external signals and cues. Specific strategies were discussed for avoiding, changing, or eliminating the signals leading to smoking, and subjects were advised to eliminate the cigarettes of least need. Rewards, target dates, and training in deep breathing and relaxation were also part of the method. Five sessions over 3 weeks were held with quit day on the ninth day; after 6 months followup, 24% of the subjects had stopped smoking.

In another study, subjects were assigned to cue extinction, self-control, or a combination of the two; cue extinction (a procedure to extinguish associations between desires for cigarettes and cues paired with previous smoking) was not as effective as were self-control techniques, with only 8% stopping smoking; self-control techniques alone achieved a quit rate of 29%, and combined techniques achieved a quit rate of 27%.

The third classification of stimulus control is deprived response performance. The technique has been used as a means of actualizing the subjects' responsibility in assuming a direct role in the quitting process. Programs have used a combination of this technique with individual counseling, covert conditioning, contingency management, relaxation, and other self-control techniques. Studies which have appeared in the literature do not provide evidence to support stimulus control as a cessation procedure; stimulus control appears to assist smokers to reduce their smoking rather than getting them to quit. Perhaps the reduced number of cigarettes take on more importance, or the cigarettes still smoked are the toughest ones to give up. Keeping a detailed account of when each cigarette is smoked and the related activities and feelings can provide the smoker with insight to the smoking habit, and this activity in turn can assist the smoker to quit, as long as the treatment also includes some type of relapse prevention and maintenance support.

Contingency Management

There is an implied contract, between the volunteer and the program, in almost all smoking cessation programs, that the client will complete questionnaires, participate in treatment, attempt to quit, and provide follow-up information. Except in a few programs, no formal contract is presented or agreed upon. Many programs collect a small deposit that is returned if the client attends treatment sessions or submits follow-up data. A number of employers have offered monetary incentives to employees who either refrain from smoking at work or quit altogether (see section on this technique). These instances are not considered to be contractual.

The purpose of contingency contracting is to emphasize the goals of the smoker while enhancing motivation through commitment. Two forms of these contracts are monetary deposit systems and social contracts with peers. The concept of social contracts has not been tested with sufficient scientific rigor.

The practice of making public statements to peers or colleagues regarding one's intention to quit smoking, however, is not uncommon to most smokers. It tends to be an accessible form of motivation on which to base hopes of cessation. Return of a money deposit is generally contingent on abstinence but sometimes is tied to reduction in the number of cigarettes smoked. Thus, the money deposit acts to reinforce cessation behavior.

In summary, contracting leads to some measure of success during treatment or until the deposit is returned. Once the contract has ended, many subjects regress unless maintenance is provided. Use of contracting as one aspect of a multicomponent program may contribute to success, but as the primary treatment, contingent contracting is limited in its application.

Systematic Desensitization and Relaxation

Desensitization was designed to strengthen responses that are incompatible with smoking. The investigators hypothesized that smoking behavior is frequently cued to anxiety and that if the prior and proximal stimuli leading to smoking were desensitized, then smoking would diminish. Other investigators suggested that subjects could be conditioned to relax as an alternative to smoking. Still others believed that reducing the stress generated by quitting would help to create positive results.

The early use of desensitization techniques in smoking control proved disappointing, with low quit rates (10% and 19% from two studies that conducted 6-month follow-ups). Relaxation training has been offered by a variety of programs, including voluntary and commerical clinics and hypnotherapists. A number of behavioral investigators have used relaxation techniques along with other treatment procedures. Such combinations reported by investigators include rapid smoking, rapid smoking and self-control, normal paced aversive smoking, smoke holding, covert sensitization, contingency contracting, self-control, stimulus control, self-monitoring and smoke aversion, and multicomponent programs. Relaxation programs by themselves do not result in smoking cessation.

Controlled studies do not support desensitization as a treatment for smoking. Although relaxation seems to make sense as a helpful procedure, insofar as nicotine has primarily stimulating effects, the smoker seeking stimulation may not find relaxation satisfying enough to replace smoking.

Restricted Environmental Stimulation Therapy (REST)

This procedure derives its rationale from evidence that a period of sensory deprivation leads to generally increased persuadability and responsiveness to external cues. The procedure facilitates openness to new information and reduced defensiveness. REST is an attitude change technique in which a subject remains in a dark, soundproof chamber in a bed for a long period, usually 24 hours. A monitor is on duty during the entire treatment session and has audio contact with the subject. In some conditions, subjects periodically hear messages concerning the dangers of cigarette smoking and methods of controlling the urge for a cigarette. Less than 24 hours of confinement is considered partial REST. Restricted environmental stimulation therapy is also called sensory deprivation.

There has been little interest in sensory deprivation as a smoking cessation method, as evidenced by only three studies reported after 1977 and only a few before that date. Some researchers maintain that REST is cost effective because it calls for little expense and minimal therapist contact, and the procedure is safe and nonadversive. REST, however, requires a special chamber or room and standby staff for a full 24 hours. It appears to be impractical for reaching and curing a large number of smokers.

Self-Control Packages

Almost all multiple smoking cessation programs include self-control procedures. Although they differ widely, three types can be distinguished. Each type can be further subdivided into programs that include aversive smoking procedures and those that do not. Simple programs are those that combine a single procedure with self-control. Coping strategy programs include as a major component coping strategies, relapse prevention, abstinence training, or anxiety management. Multiple programs combine three or more techniques.

Many multicomponent programs include smoke aversion as a way of breaking the habit and self-control to maintain nonsmoking. This combination appears to improve quit rates over smoke aversion alone, but there have been exceptions. Individualized and flexible self-management plus either rapid smoking or satiation or both aversive procedures has been found to be effective. Each smoker would have an individual coping strategy that included relaxation, deep breathing, behavioral rehearsal, covert control, contingency contracting, stimulus control and social support. This combined approach had a 47% success rate with a group of 60 subjects after 6 months.

Another combined program used nicotine fading with self-management for an improved result, but others have not fared as well. Emphasis on abstinence training usually produces good quit rates, while other programs were successful with brand fading and abstinence training, and nicotine fading and relapse prevention. Some of the very best results have been achieved with multiple treatment programs which used relapse prevention that emphasized the interacting role of coping strategies and commitment in maintaining change in addictive disorders. The program had as components: cue-produced relaxation training, commitment enhancement by reviews of the costs of smoking and the benefits of nonsmoking, and relapse prevention skill training in which subjects identified relapse situations and either role played or rethought these situations. Relapse training is claimed as effective, but requires considerable skill to implement effectively.

Some multicomponent programs prepare manuals that guide subjects in their quitting program and provide instructions on how to apply the self-management procedures. Studies on therapist-administered self-control strategies suggest the potential superiority of multicomponent behavioral approaches. Multicomponent programs remain attractive because they can deal with the multiple factors maintaining smoking as well as with the considerable individual differences among smokers.

In summary, smoking is a complex habit causally related to a variety of pharmacological, environmental, cognitive, and affective factors. Psychological factors involved in the smoking habit are central to the problems of smoking modification. The key factor in assisting smokers to break the habit rests with the maintenance phase rather than in the initial treatment. Self-management of the smoking problem is valid because the smoker relies less on the leader or therapist and more on himself or herself, leading to a more lasting change because success in quitting is self-attributed rather than credited to other sources.

High Risk Populations

The majority of workplace smoking program participants have been young, from middle or upper socioeconomic levels, and in occupations that do not place them at increased health risk. Although smoking cessation efforts should continue with such populations, an argument can be made for focusing efforts on persons at very high risk for cancer, cardiovascular disease, or respiratory disease; these diseases are the major causes of excess morbidity and mortality due to cigarette smoking. Given limited resources, it should be more cost effective to direct intervention primarily toward those persons most likely to develop disease. Three overlapping approaches have been used to reach the following high risk smokers in the workplace. blue-collar male workers, workers at risk due to occupational hazards, and persons predisposed to disease because of other factors besides smoking (obesity, hypertension, etc.).

Few worksite programs have been offered by firms employing primarily male blue-collar workers, even though such groups have higher than average smoking rates. Although there is little or no documentation of the reasons for this inconsistency, it may be due to mistaken beliefs among health professionals that such individuals would be less likely to participate in or follow through with a smoking modification program. In reality, some researchers have found that blue-collar workers may be at least as interested in quitting smoking as others in the general population. Resistance on the part of some labor unions may constitute another reason for fewer programs conducted in blue-collar workplaces.

Research on worksite smoking programs with blue-collar workers has revealed that although outcomes of programs were comparable with other worksite programs, relatively low compliance rates and possible failure to recruit a high percentage of smokers may have caused the apparently less favorable outcome. Perhaps a different intervention approach is needed for blue-collar workers, one that does not require much devotion of time and effort, and one that tailors materials and tasks to be socioculturally appropriate.

Little systematic research with smokers in jobs that place them at risk because of occupational hazards has been reported. For instance, asbestos workers are at high risk for respiratory disease, and workers who smoke increase their risk synergistically. A study was made of a smoking reduction program for former asbestos workers that involved incorporating antismoking advice into regularly scheduled appointments with company doctors, pairing written self-help materials with feedback on physical status, and offering individual smoking cessation counseling. Over a 4-year period, this relatively low-cost intervention was associated with a 30% reduction in the proportion of employees who reported being smokers.

The most extensive no-smoking program involving high risk occupations was conducted by the Johns-Manville asbestos company. In addition to a smoking ban throughout the workplace and a company policy of no longer hiring new employees who smoke, Johns-Manville launched an intensive anti-smoking campaign at 14 company sites. This program involved an educational campaign coordinated with Smoke-Enders cessation clinics, and the institution of a companywide smoking ban. Although systematic, published reports of this program were not available, reported participation rates of

15%-20% in the cessation clinics and an approximately 75% posttreatment quit rate among participants were attained. In the only controlled study to date of worksite intervention in high risk worker populations, the effects of physician stop-smoking advice on asbestos-exposed naval shipyard workers were measured. Surprisingly, subjects who had abnormal pulmonary function tests did not have higher cessation rates than workers with normal function tests.

The third approach to reaching high risk participants has been to conduct comprehensive health screenings to identify individuals at risk for the development of chronic disease. It has been found that high risk people in intervention programs were more successful at quitting smoking than similar subjects in controls.

Multiple Risk Factor Reduction Programs

A number of organizations have offered smoking cessation programs as part of employee wellness or lifestyle-modification programs. Such programs typically focus on achieving modifications in several risk areas in addition to cigarette smoking, such as obesity, elevated cholesterol levels, hypertension, and a sedentary life style. Some programs also include components on stress management and modifying Type A behavior. Almost all programs include an initial health screening to identify risk factors, but subsequently there is a considerable divergence in approaches. Some programs focus solely on high risk participants; others invite all employees to participate regardless of risk status. There is also considerable variation in how smoking programs are implemented, with some programs holding separate meetings for smokers, and others including information on smoking modification as part of their general wellness program.

The concept of providing smoking modification services as part of a more general lifestyle program is appealing. Stopping smoking can be seen as one aspect of adopting a more healthy lifestyle, and other program components such as increased levels of exercise may reinforce smoking abstinence. Many smokers, particularly women, are concerned about potential weight gain as a result of smoking cessation, and such programs can address these concerns.

There are also potential disadvantages with multiple risk factor reduction programs. They may be difficult to implement because staff expertise is required in multiple areas and because some risk factors, such as smoking, may not be relevant for all participants. In addition, multiple risk factor reduction programs must present a large amount of complex information, usually in a limited time, and consequently the amount of attention devoted to a particular risk factor such as smoking must often be less than is the case in single-topic programs.

Two main types of multiple risk factor reduction programs have involved smoking cessation. The first were large-scale clinical trials for prevention of coronary heart disease, conducted by WHO in Belgium and Great Britain. The trials were conducted solely in industrial settings, were well-designed, and collected multiple dependent variables, including indices of overall health risk or morbidity and mortality statistics. The other main type of multiple risk factor reduction program that has been developed is exemplified by worksite wellness programs developed by large firms for their workers. Examples include the STAYWELL program on Control Data Corporation, the Live for Life program of Johnson & Johnson, and programs offered by IBM, Campbell Soup Company, and Ford Motor Company. Unfortunately, the outcomes of almost all industry-sponsored programs reported to date are difficult to interpret, due to varying methods of reporting results, difficulties in following subjects, and lack of objective measures of smoking status.

Cessation rates in multiple risk factor reduction programs in worksites have ranged from 7%-33% at followup. Many of these rates are lower than those typically reported in other worksite smoking studies, and are not consistently better than comparison conditions in controlled studies. Interpretation of these data is problematic because of the lack of direct comparisons with smoking-cessation-only intervention programs, because subjects with multiple risk factors may be more recalcitrant than other subjects, and because these risk factor reduction programs tend to be ongoing programs rather than one-shot smoking clinics.

REFERENCES

1. Grabowski, John, and Sharon M. Hall, Eds. *Pharmacological Adjuncts in Smoking Cessation* (NIDA Research Monograph 53). U. S. Department of Health and Human Services, Public Health Service. Washington, D.C: Superintendent of Documents, U.S. Government Printing Office, 1985. DHHS Publication No. (ADM) 85–1333.

2. *Clinical Opportunities For Smoking Intervention: A Guide For the Busy Physican*. U.S. Department of Health and Human Services, Public Health Service. Washington, DC: Superintendent of Documents, U.S. Government Printing Office, 1986. NIH Publication No. 86–2178.

Self-Help Books and Other Self-Help Materials

American Cancer Society. *I Quit Kit*.

American Lung Association:
Freedom From Smoking in 20 Days, 63 pp.
In Control (2 hrs), video, MMI Video Inc., Chicago.
A Lifetime of Freedom From Smoking, 28 pp.

Amit, Z., E.A. Sutherland, and A.Weiner. *Stop Smoking for Good*. Walker and Co., New York, 1976, 222 pp.

Burton, D. and G. Wohl. *The Joy of Quitting. How to Help Young People Stop Smoking*. Collier Books, New York, 1979, 100 pp.

Casewit, C. *Quit Smoking*. Para Research, Inc., Rockport, MA, 1983, 144 pp.

Danaher, B.G. and E. Lichtenstein. *Become an Ex-Smoker*. Prentice-Hall, Inc., Engelwood Cliffs, NJ, 1978, 237 pp.

Ferguson, T. *The Smoker's Book of Health: How to Keep Yourself Healthier and Cut Your Smoking Risk*. Putnam Publishing Group, New York, 1987, 224 pp.

Holland, G. and H. Weiss. *Quit Smoking in 30 Days*. Bantam Books, Des Plaines, IL, 1984, 64 pp.

National Cancer Institute:
Helping Smokers Quit Kit
Quit for Good Kit contains *Quit It* and *For Good* pamphlets.
Helping Smokers Quit Kit for pharmacists.
Clearing the Air
You've Kicked the Smoking Habit— For Good!

Ogle, J. *The Stop Smoking Diet*. Evans and Co., New York, 1981, 168 pp.

Olshavsky, R.W. *No More Butts—A Psychologist's Approach to Quitting Cigarettes*. Indiana University Press, Bloomington, IN, 1977, 181 pp.

Pomerleau, O.F. and C.S. Pomerleau. *Break the Smoking Habit: A Behavioral Program for Giving Up Cigarettes*. Research Press, Champaign, IL, 1977, 141 pp.

Rogers, J. *You Can Stop. A SmokEnder Approach to Quitting Smoking and Sticking to It*. Simon and Schuster, New York, 1977, 191 pp.

Stanford University. *Quit Kit*.

U.S. Department of Health, Education, and Welfare, Public Health Service, and National Clearinghouse for Smoking and Health. *Smoker's Self-Testing Kit*. PHS Publ. No. 1904, U.S. Government Printing Office, Washington, DC, 1969. Also publishes the *Teenage Self-Test*.

U.S. Office on Smoking and Health. *Helping Smokers Quit* (pamphlet); *Calling it Quits: The Latest Advice on How to Give Up Cigarettes* (pamphlet).

7

Program Implementation and Outcomes

This final chapter discusses promotion and recruitment of smokers, program characteristics, outcomes of programs, and organizational characteristics influencing the program results. Maintenance of smoking cessation, characteristics of successful quitters and backsliders, relapse situations, and maintenance strategies conclude the chapter.

IMPLEMENTATION OF WORKSITE SMOKING PROGRAMS

Promotion and Recruitment

The initial contact with a workplace can prove critical to the success of a project. It is generally recommended that the initial meeting be with the chief executive of the organization. Although this officer typically does not coordinate the program, support from top-level management appears to be important in program recruitment and implementation. Another method of enhancing participation and organizational involvement is the formation of a steering committee composed of key representatives from both labor and management. Employees should perceive that the program is voluntary and that they have input into its implementation. Steering committees of this type may be particularly important in large worksites with unionized employees. Management support appears to be quite important to the success of the committee.

Upon securing permission to offer a program, it is helpful to conduct a brief workplace needs assessment. The survey can be used to determine: (1) the number and characteristics of smokers in the workplace, (2) the number of smokers potentially interested in participating, and (3) preferences concerning the types of programs that might be offered (for example, self-help versus group meetings; abstinence versus reduced smoking) and the most convenient times for meetings to be scheduled.

During the recruitment phase, information about the program should come from a variety of sources, such as posters, memos, and brochures. Advertising experts recommend providing multiple exposures to a "product" (here, the smoking program) to promote attitude change and to convince participants to take action regarding the product. Promotional materials should include information about the cost of a program, stress that participation is voluntary and individual results are confidential, and counter possible misconceptions (such as having to quit after the first session, or losing one's job if smoking is not stopped). It is helpful if at least one memo or announcement comes from top management. At this stage, human resources or personnel directors can be extremely useful in suggesting the best ways to promote the program in their particular setting. Involving the local media may also increase the credibility of the program, as well as provide no-cost advertising for both the program and the worksite.

Prior to the actual implementation of a smoking program, some programs prepare workplaces for health-behavior change. These preparatory procedures have ranged from prescreening health exams to the initiation of smoking restrictions. Warnings of the impending restrictions with indications of the "target restriction date" allow workers to prepare for changes, such as by joining available programs. Although empirically untested, these recruitment procedures may help to convince employees to join smoking programs.

Program Characteristics

The advantages of occupational smoking control programs discussed earlier do not automatically or necessarily occur. Programs must be made convenient. Higher participation rates are usually found in programs that offer time off from work. Time off from work for participation can be a double-edged sword, however; it may increase the number of smokers who participate primarily to be excused from their work areas, and it may also create demands among nonsmoking employees for time off to attend other health-related activities. Generally, the benefits of conducting programs during working hours outweigh the potential costs, and if management is not willing to grant time off from work, it may at least be possible to negotiate time sharing between employee and employer to make possible attendance at the program. Investigators should also be aware of difficulties involved in scheduling group meetings in workplaces where employees work rotating shifts, such as at hospitals.

In addition to being convenient, programs should be attractive to participants. For example, allowing smokers to choose the type of program (such as nicotine fading versus aversive smoking), the form of intervention (self-help manuals versus group meetings), and the type of group leader (health professional versus peer group member) may be helpful in attracting and retaining participants. Different components of a comprehensive program, such as physician advice, no-smoking policies, stop-smoking contests, or group meetings, may be mutually reinforcing. While these suggestions await empirical verification, providing smokers with a variety of choices should serve to increase participation rates.

Finally, feedback on progress may serve to increase the magnitude of behavior change. For example, participants can be provided with frequent feedback on carbon monoxide levels as they reduce their smoking. Charts displaying the weekly progress of different groups can be posted in employee lunch areas or lounges. Periodic progress reports to department supervisors may be helpful. To avoid stigmatizing particular workers, public feedback should be provided on progress by the group, rather than by individuals.

There are a number of problems in conducting worksite smoking modification groups that should be avoided, or at least anticipated. Group composition is one such sensitive issue; mixing high-ranking executives with production workers can almost eliminate group discussion. However, this may depend on the firm's tradition of interaction among workers of different levels, on the skills of the group leaders, and so forth. Scheduling difficulties can arise in settings where employees rotate shifts or travel frequently, or where meeting rooms are scarce or distant from work areas. One must also be sensitive to negativism or complaining, which can become contagious; the group's focus must be kept positive. A positive perspective is particularly important when conducting competition or incentive interventions in which certain individuals or groups must "lose." A more optimistic perspective that can be used to encourage participants is that everyone can win something by changing their smoking habits, so there are no losers.

Finally, the concept of stopping smoking as a "journey" can be quite helpful. On their journey, persons may experience temporary setbacks or detours (relapses), but this should not prevent them from reaching their destination (abstinence). The presence of an ongoing program that makes it easy to try different options or to recycle a procedure can serve to reinforce this concept and to improve long-term results.

OUTCOME OF STOP-SMOKING PROGRAMS

Organizational Characteristics and Other Factors

Conducting outcome research in worksite settings involves a number of unique factors that may mediate or interact with program success. The organizational characteristics that may mediate program success include: size of workplace; current workplace smoking policies; degree of management support for program; history of health promotion efforts in the workplace; sex ratio of employees; job stability and turnover rate; union-management relations; percent of smokers in the worksite; growth oriented vs. consolidating climate of organization; rank and sociometric standing of primary contact person; and socioeconomic level of employees. Although this list is certainly not exhaustive, investigators should consider these factors when designing and conducting worksite smoking programs.

Few of these variables have been addressed in workplace smoking studies. Researchers who have conducted similar multilevel smoking cessation programs in several different organizations have reported substantially lower participation in large firms, a finding consistent with worksite weight-loss programs. Some studies have yielded data that suggest that highest cessation rates are found at smaller worksites. These trends, taken together, suggest that different intervention patterns and different participation routes need to be developed for large firms. The problem may be one of implementation, not design. Company policy regarding vesting responsibility in division leadership may be a critical variable.

In terms of current worksite smoking policies as a variable, it is important to emphasize that smoking cessation groups are but one way to influence rates of workplace cigarette smoking.

Although there have certainly been more reports on cessation programs than on other approaches to occupational smoking control, evaluations of alternative procedures are beginning to appear. Studies have been made of the effects of no-smoking signs and requests not to smoke; these studies indicate that the posting of no-smoking signs and establishment of nonsmoking areas temporarily reduce smoking rates, but that active enforcement of such policies is needed to produce substantial or lasting reduction in smoking behavior. One caveat to be kept in mind in evaluating the effects of workplace smoking restrictions is that workers may "compensate" by smoking more during breaks and after work. Evaluations of effectiveness of smoking restrictions should therefore assess smoking rates during both work and nonwork hours and include objective measures of smoking exposure.

Smoking modification efforts can be divided into three categories: smoking control, the limiting or restricting of smoking to designated areas; smoking discouragement, the educational efforts to encourage people to stop smoking; and smoking cessation, the more formal treatment programs. It should be noted that worksite smoking cessation programs operate most effectively when they are offered together with workplace smoking control and discouragement efforts; this hypothesis is highly testable, but has yet to be experimentally investigated.

The potential to use work environment modifications to aid smoking cessation, including restricting smoking, removing cigarette machines, and altering work rules or situations that promote smoking, make the workplace more than simply a location for cessation intervention. The elimination of environmental supports for smoking, alteration of the smoker's self-image, changing the perception of the smoker among peers, and revising the social norms about smoking in the workplace may all provide a powerful motivation for the smoker to quit and support the successful maintenance of cessation. These changes in the workplace environment and attitudes may be more important than the components of the behavioral intervention used to get workers to quit, and experimental verification of the impact of these changes would provide a useful guide for the structuring of future comprehensive worksite intervention programs. Because it would probably be unlikely that researchers would gain access to experimental manipulation of some of the more controversial aspects of guidelines, such as hiring policies and penalties for smoking, opportunities that may arise to study such changes in uncontrolled research would be worth pursuing.

Few data have been collected on other variables listed previously, the organizational characteristics that may mediate program success; research on workplace smoking programs should at least provide descriptive information to determine how these variables affect program success. The fit between organizational and program characteristics has been neglected in past occupational smoking control research.

LONG-TERM MAINTENANCE OF SMOKING CESSATION

The key to a successful cessation program is maintenance support. Almost any kind of treatment, including a control condition, generates some quitters. Initial success rates as high as 80%–100% have been reported; however, during the first 4 months, a high number of successes become recidivists, and during the next 8 months, other ex-smokers return to smoking. As long-term follow-ups have shown, some people return to smoking even after one year. It has been found that a 33% follow-up quit rate in smoking cessation is good. In the mid-1970s, researchers began paying attention to maintenance, and some reported improved success rates.

What Characterizes Quitters and Recidivists?

With a few exceptions, early studies indicated that success in giving up smoking was inversely related to the average daily amount smoked, and directly related to age of starting smoking. Success in smoking cessation was also related to a spouse's smoking habits, and some studies related smoking friends to difficulty in quitting. Other studies found no such relationships. There is an extensive literature on the prediction of cessation and long-term maintenance.

Researchers have analyzed profiles of successful quitters and recidivists who had participated in the Smoking Control Research Project (SCRP). Of 252 male subjects, 33% initially stopped smoking, with the quit rate declining to 20% by the 4-month and 1-year follow-up times. A cluster analysis reduced 101 variables to 10 meaningful and relatively independent "clusters." The 252 subjects were scored on the 5 most salient clusters resulting in 12 profile types.

The first cluster selected was "personal adjustment," or contentment, in such areas as work, achievement, sex, and social situations. This was the individual's expressed confidence, security, or satisfaction with various aspects of his or her life. The second cluster combined chronic illness and anxiety, recent respiratory illnesses, and use of psychiatric care. Perceptions of smoking made up the third cluster. Low scores on this dimension represented greater belief in the health danger of cigarettes. The fourth cluster related to the degree to which smoking was internalized and included the habitual and addictive dimensions of smoking. "Smoking affect," the fifth cluster, included concepts of negative and positive affect.

The 12 profile types were created without regard to outcome in smoking cessation. Each type was then examined for success and recidivism. Four profile types contained 60% of the continuing successes but only 20% of the recidivists. These types all had good adjustment, low illness and anxiety, and low chronic, habitual, and addictive smoking scores. The type that contained a good success rate throughout the study possessed all the characteristics normally associated with high probability of success; besides having the motivation and proper cognitive frame of mind, they were not hindered by personal problems or by an overwhelming need to smoke. The next three types, which contained fewer successes, where characterized by average adjustment, high chronic illness and anxiety, and high chronic, habitual, and addictive smoking.

Although there were few similarities among types high in recidivism, two kinds of recidivists could be distinguished. The first showed poor personal adjustment, which may have accounted for their return to smoking. The second kind of recidivist showed good adjustment but scored high in two of the three smoking factors. Thus some were high in habitual and addictive smoking and affect smoking, but not perception of smoking dangers; others were high in habitual and addictive smoking and perception but not affect; and some were high on affect and perception but not habitual and addictive smoking.

When the remaining five clusters not used in the typology were examined, "smoking environment" (the smoking habits of the spouse and patterns of smoking with friends) appeared to differentiate continuing successes from recidivists. Successes tended to have smoking environment scores more conducive to quitting. Moreover, once the subject had stopped, the probability of continued abstinence was greatly increased if there was less smoking on the part of his or her friends and spouse.

Successes as a group scored higher in personal adjustment and lower in habitual and addictive smoking and smoking affect. They also had a somewhat lower incidence of chronic illness and anxiety. In addition, successes had a more negative perception of smoking than did recidivists.

Studies have also been made of the tobacco withdrawal syndrome; the syndrome is characterized by changes in the EEG and cardiovascular functions, by decrements in psychomotor performance, and by weight gain. Subjective symptoms of irritability, anxiety, inability to concentrate, and disturbances of arousal are characteristic of tobacco users in withdrawal, and intense cravings for tobacco are universally reported. Withdrawal symptoms vary in intensity and duration, and researchers have advised that interventions that directly attack withdrawal symptoms need to be developed and evaluated. Manipulation of patients' expectations or attributions of withdrawal symptoms might be a route to the reduction of the symptoms' severity.

The SCRP study developed three other items to measure previous experience with smoking cessation, ease and success in stopping, and expectation of success in giving up smoking. Perhaps related to their favorable orientation toward cessation, continuing successes had more often found it "easy" to quit in previous attempts, compared to recidivists. In regard to differences in expectation of future smoking, relatively more successes than recidivists thought that they would not be smoking in one year. There seems to be a subgroup of persons who do not consider quitting very difficult, who are confident that they can stop smoking, and who are, in turn, most likely to succeed in an organized withdrawal program, perhaps because they are already on the verge of quitting.

Relapse Situations

Studies have found that the majority of relapse situations involved social pressure to smoke. Causes for relapse fell into three categories: social pressures, coping with negative emotional states, and coping with interpersonal conflict. The primary setting for smoking relapse was the home, followed by the work environment, restaurants and bars, and parties. The evening was most often cited as the time of relapse. A single slip often resulted in total recidivism. Effective maintenance requires that the smoker be taught cognitive recognition and behavior analysis as well as coping responses to relapse stimuli.

Good self-image, optimism, and a good feeling of self-satisfaction characterized success for SCRP subjects; these people were socially outgoing, had good relationships within the family, and responded positively to concern about their smoking. They expressed confidence in their self-control and rational behavior. Since they accepted themselves realistically and trusted others, they were not overly afraid of failure. More willing to commit themselves to a goal, they were more able to achieve the goal.

Typically, in the home situation of the recidivist, the spouse smoked and did not give the subject much support in his or her quitting. Recidivists did not emphasize the importance of smoking as a tension reducer but spoke more often of the physical gratification derived. It is important to note that these subjects were able to stop smoking, if only temporarily. Clearly, however, these subjects were unable to maintain abstinence without continued pressure, whether in the form of an organized program, an environment that emphasized the health dangers of smoking, or aid from their spouses or close associates. Without such outside supports, the typical recidivist, who lacks the inner resources to cope with the loss of cigarettes, has virtually nothing to prevent him or her from resuming the habit.

MAINTENANCE STRATEGIES FOR SMOKING CESSATION

Maintenance is viewed by some as a gradual transition away from cessation. Maintenance strategies, including social support, coping skills, and cognitive restructuring, have been identified as necessary. Social support is based on a notion that a group or close companions can provide enough support or influence to help the individual sustain the motivation to continue nonsmoking. Coping skills are required to help the new nonsmoker deal with the discomfort of cigarette deprivation, in developing substitute responses to replace smoking, in learning to recognize and modify the cues to smoke, and in altering the consequences of smoking. Cognitive restructuring involves changing attitudes and self-perceptions related to smoking behavior.

SPECIAL ISSUES RELEVANT TO WORKSITE PROGRAMS

Social Support

One frequently cited reason for having smoking modification programs in the workplace is the potential for using peer and environmental support for nonsmoking. It has been argued that peer support has important, long-lasting effects on the outcome of stop-smoking efforts, and there have been several calls for increased study of the role of social support in smoking modification. There are also correlational findings that suggest the importance of social support to successful smoking cessation efforts.

Given this background, it is surprising that a large-scale correlational study of occupational settings found that the degree of perceived support from coworkers was *inversely* related to smoking status. Among workers with low job stress levels, ex-smokers reported lower levels of support than did current smokers. There was no relationship between social support and smoking status for workers with high job stress levels. More recent studies have noted a complex relationship between social support and outcome of worksite smoking modification programs. Using a measure that produced a score for both supportive and nonsupportive social interactions, researchers found that the presence of smoking-related negative social interactions was inversely related to treatment success. The presence of positive social support, frequently the target of social support interventions, was not related to outcome.

Social support procedures, such as a buddy system and inclusion of nonsmoking coworkers or family members in treatment sessions, have been part of a variety of workplace programs; unfortunately, it is impossible to evaluate the contribution of social support in these studies because of the number of other intervention strategies also used. It has been noted, however, that incentive programs that included spouses were more successful than those that did not.

The few workplace smoking studies that attempted to experimentally manipulate social support levels have produced discouraging results. Social support/social skills training programs including buddy systems with health education and cognitive-behavioral stress management procedures as ways to improve long-term effectiveness of nicotine-fading cessation programs were unsuccessful; subjects in the social support/social skills condition had relapsed significantly more than those in other conditions. Additionally, consumer satisfaction ratings revealed that subjects liked social support/social skills programs less well than other options. Evidently, factors such as social support, theoretically assumed to enhance treatment, may actually reduce the effectiveness of a treatment program.

Studies evaluating the effects of adding a coworker support component to a multicomponent treatment program offering subjects the options of abstinence or controlled smoking found that the addition of coworker support did not improve treatment outcome, and that subjects did not find the social support condition as credible as the basic program. Therefore, the inclusion of existing social support procedures has not been found to enhance outcome in workplace smoking modification programs, basically because the issue is more complex than previously believed.

Selected References

Basic References

Health Consequences of Involuntary Smoking: A Report of the Surgeon General. U.S. Department of Health and Human Services, Public Health Service. Washington, DC: Superintendent of Documents, U.S. Government Printing Office, 1986. 359 pp. DHHS (CDC)87-8398. pp. 7, 21–28, 132–147, 164–169, 181–198, 229–252, 265–308.

Health Consequences of Smoking. Cancer and Chronic Lung Disease in the Workplace: A Report of the Surgeon General. U.S. Department of Health and Human Services, Public Health Service. Washington, DC: Superintendent of Documents, U.S. Government Printing Office, 1985. 542 pp. DHHS(PHS)85-50207. pp. 11–17, 23–38, 48–53, 477–506.

Passive Smoking in the Workplace: Selected Issues. Staff paper prepared by the Special Projects Office of the Health Program, Office of Technology Assessment: U.S. Congress, 1986, 70 pp. (NTIS PB86-217627). pp. 1–2, 4–5, 8–59.

Schwartz, Jerome L. *Review and Evaluation of Smoking Cessation Methods: The United States and Canada, 1978–1985.* Division of Cancer Prevention and Control, National cancer Institute; U.S. Department of Health and Human Services, Public Health Service, National Institutes of Health. NIH Publication 87-2940, 1987. 200 pp.

Effects of Smoking on Work Performance

Atkinson, A.B., and T.W. Meade. "Methods and preliminary findings in assessing the economic and health services consequences of smoking, with particular reference to lung cancer," *Journal of the Royal Statistical Society* 136, 297–312, 1974. (NTIS HRP-0011060/1)

Breidenbach, Steven T., James L. Arnold, and Norman W. Heimstra. *The Effects of Smoking on Time Estimation Performance.* Vermillion, SD: University of South Dakota, 1976. 69 pp. (NTIS AD-A047744/8)

Burse, Richard L., Ralph F. Goldman, Elliot Danforth, Jr., Edward S. Horton, and Ethan A.H. Sims. *Effects of Cigarette Smoking on Body Weight, Energy Expenditure, Appetite and Endocrine Function.* Natick, MA: Army Research Inst. of Environmental Medicine, 1982. 29 pp. (NTIS AD-A114213/2)

Conway, T.L., and T.A. Cronan. *Smoking and Physical Fitness Among Navy Shipboard Personnel.* San Diego, CA: Naval Health Research Center, 1986. 21 pp. (NTIS AD-A180160/4/XAB)

Dembert, M.L., G.J. Beck, J.F. Jekel, and L.W. Mooney. "Relations of smoking and diving experience to pulmonary function among U.S. Navy divers," *Undersea Biomedical Research* 11(3), 299–304, 1984. (NTIS AD-A164481/4/XAB)

Fine, Bernard J., and John L. Kobrick. *Cigarette Smoking, Field-Dependence and Contrast Sensitivity*. Natick, MA: Army Research Inst. of Environmental Medicine, 1986. 24 pp. (NTIS AD-A173450/8/XAB)

Gibson, Richard S., and William F. Moroney. *A Limited Review of the Effect of Cigarette Smoking on Performance with Emphasis on Aviation*. Pensacola, FL: Naval Aerospace Medical Inst., 1972. 12 pp. (NTIS AD-754 421)

Heimstra, Norman W. *The Effects of Smoking on Peripheral Movement Detection and Time Estimation Performance*. Vermillion, SD: University of South Dakota, 1977. 9 pp. (NTIS AD-A052693/9)

Hirsch, G.L., D.Y. Sue, K. Wasserman, T.E. Robinson, and J.E. Hansen. "Immediate effects of cigarette smoking on cardiorespiratory responses to exercise," *Journal of Applied Physiology* 58(6), 1975–1981, 1985. (NIOSH-00149470)

Kozak, J.T. "Contribution of smoking habit to work incapacity," *Bulletin of the Industrial Union Against Tuberculosis* 59(1–2), 48–49, 1984. (NIOSH-00153741)

Mertens, Henry W., Jess M. McKenzie, and E. Arnold Higgins. *Some Effects of Smoking Withdrawal on Complex Performance and Physiological Responses*. Washington, DC: Federal Aviation Administration, 1983. 18 pp. (NTIS AD-A126551/1)

Millis, R.M. *Review of the Scientific Literature and Preparation of an Annotated Bibliography on Effects of Cigarette Smoking and Nicotine on Human Performance*. Volume 1. Washington, DC: Associate Consultants, Inc., 1986. 187 pp. (NTIS AD-A186805/8/XAB)

Millis, R.M. *Review of the Scientific Literature and Preparation of an Annotated Bibliography on Effects of Cigarette Smoking and Nicotine on Human Performance*. Volume 2. Washington, DC: Associate Consultants, Inc., 1985. 156 pp. (NTIS AD-A186806/6/XAB)

Parkes, K.R. "Smoking as a moderator of the relationship between affective state and absence from work," *Journal of Applied Psychology* 68(4), 698–708, 1983. (NIOSH-00138526)

Scoughton, Craig R., and Norman W. Heimstra. *The Effects of Smoking on Peripheral Movement Detection*. Vermillion, SD: University of South Dakota, 1973. 50 pp. (NTIS AD-778 928/2)

Van Tuinen, M., and G. Land. "Smoking and excess sick leave in a department of health," *Journal of Occupational Medicine* 28(1), 33–35, 1986. (NIOSH-00157740)

Yuste, P.C., and M.L. de Guevara. "The influence of smoking on work accidents. Statistical survey," *Medicine y Seguridad del Trabajo* 21(84), 38–46, 1973. (NIOSH-00104258)

Quitting Smoking

Baker, Leonard S. "To help schools combat smoking," *American Education* 14(8), 18–23, Oct. 1978.

Dubren, Ron. "Evaluation of a televised stop-smoking clinic," *Public Health Reports* 92(1), 81–84, Jan.–Feb. 1977.

Ferguson, Tom. "The guilt-free guide to a smoke-free life: Finally, a stop-smoking method that doesn't nag, pressure, threaten or blame," *Modern Maturity* 32(1), 76–77, 80–81, 83–86, 91, Feb.–Mar. 1989.

Krasnegor, Norman A. *The Behavioral Aspects of Smoking*. National Institute on Drug Abuse, Rockville, MD: 1979. 199 pp. Research Monograph 26. DHEW/PUB/ADM-79/882; NIDA/RD-79/31. (NTIS PB80-118755)

Milligan, Robert C., and W. Bernard Suttake. *Developing Smoking Cessation Classes with Major Community Involvement*. Paper, 1975 Annual Meeting, American Public Health Association. 14 pp. (NTIS HRP-0006777/7)

"Smoking cessation: The best ways to kick the deadliest, most expensive addiction," *Health Letter* (Public Citizen Health Research Group) 4(10), 1–7, 1988.

"Smoking cessation, Part II: How the government, the medical establishment, and insurers have neglected America's deadliest, most costly addiction," *Health Letter* (Public Citizen Health Research Group) 4(11), 6–9, 1988.

"Smoking cessation update," *Health Letter* (Public Citizen Health Research Group) 4(12), 11, 1988.

Health Effects of Smoking

Adverse Health Effects of Smoking and the Occupational Environment (Current Intelligence Bulletin 31). National Institute for Occupational Safety and Health, Cincinnati, OH: 1979. 16 pp. Report NIOSH-79-122. (NTIS PB83-245845/XAB)

Bibliography on Smoking and Health (Since 1960). Informatics General Corp., Rockville, MD: 1983, 580 pp. DHHS/PUB/PHS-83-50196; PHS/BS-45. (NTIS PB83-213215)

Cigarette Smoking: 1970–February 1986 (Citations from the NTIS Data Base). National Technical Information Service, Springfield, VA: 1986, 268 pp. (NTIS PB86-859550/XAB)

Culliton, Barbara J. "Cancer board attacks tobacco," *Science* 243(4893), 889, Feb. 17, 1989.

Directory of On-Going Research in Smoking and Health, 1982. Public Health Service, Rockville, MD: 1982. 456 pp. (NTIS PB83-210435)

Gerstein, Dean R., and Peter K. Levison. *Reduced Tar and Nicotine Cigarettes: Smoking Behavior and Health.* National Research Council, Washington, DC: 1982. 62 pp. ISBN 0-309-03246-0. (NTIS PB83-158956)

The Health Consequences of Smoking for Women: A Report of the Surgeon General. Public Health Service, Rockville, MD: 1980. 367 pp. (NTIS HRP-0902628/7)

Martell, Edward A. "Tobacco radioactivity and cancer in smokers," *American Scientist* 63(4), 404–412, 1975.

Ochsner, Alton. "The health menace of tobacco," *American Scientist* 59(2), 246–252, 1971.

Smokeless Cigarettes

"Drugs help smokers in quitting," *Knight-Ridder Newspapers,* Jan. 11, 1989.

"Pardon me, can I bum a nicotine delivery system?" *NY Times,* p. 4E, Dec. 11, 1988.

"R.J. Reynolds pulls smokeless cigarette from test markets," *Associated Press Wire Services,* Mar. 1, 1989.

"Smokers stubbing out 'smokeless' cigarette," *Associated Press Wire Services,* Dec. 14, 1988.

"U.S. health officials try to get 'smokeless' cigarette banned," *Los Angeles Times,* Dec. 4, 1988.

Addictive Nature of Tobacco

"Koop says FDA should regulate tobacco because it is addictive,", *Combined Wire Services,* July 30, 1988.

State No-Smoking Laws

Axel-Lute, Paul. *Legislation Regulating Smoking Areas: A Selective, Annotated Bibliography Through June 1978*. Bureau of Health Education, Atlanta, GA: 1976. 24 pp. HHS/CDC/CHPE-82-0043. (NTIS PB82-256199)

"All fired up over smoking," *Time,* pp. 64–69, 71–72, 75, Apr. 18, 1988.

"Anti-smoking groups fight pre-emptive laws," *Christian Science Monitor,* Feb. 19, 1989.

"Man quits over smoke, is eligible for benefits," *Associated Press Wire Services,* Dec. 28, 1988.

"Now where there's smoke, there's ire," *Hartford Courant* (Business Weekly Section), p. 20, Aug. 22, 1988.

State Legislation on Smoking and Health—1981. Centers for Disease Control, Atlanta, GA: 1982. 95 pp. HHS/CDC/CHPE-83-182. (NTIS PB83-168773)

"State smoking law seen as working," *Middletown (CT) Press,* p. 12, Sept. 21, 1988.

Other Countries

Hazarika, Sanjoy. "Fighting smoking, India to ban tobacco ads," *NY Times,* p. 22, Aug. 14, 1988.

Benefits of Quitting

"Kicking the habit," *Vogue,* p. 496, Sept. 1988.

"Older smokers still helped by quitting," *Science News* 134(22), 342, Nov. 26, 1988.

"Study finds it's never too late to quit," *Associated Press,* Nov. 24, 1988.

Federal Legislation Regulating Smoking

14 CFR Parts 121, 135 (Smoking During Aircraft Flights): FAA requires that the no-smoking sign be turned on at all times during commercial flights with origin and destination in the U.S. that are scheduled to be 2 hours or less in duration. Effective Apr. 23, 1988. (Fed Reg, p. 12358, Apr. 13, 1988)

14 CFR Part 252 (Smoking During Aircraft Flights): CAB adopts new rules to ban smoking on small aircraft and to ban cigar and pipe smoking on all flights. Regulations also retain current rules requiring fully functional ventilating systems and discouraging airlines from sandwiching nonsmokers between two smoking sections, and rejects proposals to ban smoking on short flights or to require special provisions for passengers specially sensitive to smoke. Effective July 20, 1984, adopted June 1, 1984. (Fed Reg, p. 25408, June 20, 1984)

14 CFR Part 252 (Smoking During Aircraft Flights): CAB republishes the requirement that airlines ensure that if a no-smoking section is placed between two smoking sections, the nonsmokers are not unreasonably burdened. Effective Sept. 9, 1983. (Fed Reg, p. 36093, Aug. 9, 1983)

14 CFR Part 101–120 (Smoking in Government Buildings): GSA prohibits smoking in certain areas of buildings. Regulations intend to provide a "reasonably smoke-free environment in certain areas for those working and visiting in GSA-controlled buildings." Effective Apr. 16, 1979. (Fed Reg, p. 22464, Apr. 16, 1979)

14 CFR Part 252 (Smoking During Aircraft Flights): CAB requires segregation of cigar and pipe smokers on air carriers. Requires no-smoking area for each class of service and for charter service. No-smoking area must consist of at least 2 rows of seats, and a sufficient number of seats in the no-smoking areas of the aircraft must be made available to accommodate all persons wishing to sit in those areas. Provides for the expansion of no-smoking areas to meet passenger demands, and provides special provisions insuring that if a no-smoking section is placed between smoking sections, that the non-smoking passengers are not "unreasonably burdened." Effective Feb. 23, 1979. (Fed Reg, p. 5071, Jan. 29, 1979)

32 CFR Part 203 (Smoking in Government Buildings): DOD publishes its policy in prohibiting smoking in DOD buildings and facilities. Effective Aug. 18, 1977. (Fed Reg, p. 57123, Nov. 1, 1977)

Richman, L.A., and B.S. Jonas. *Final Report on the Impact of Anti-Smoking Policies in the Federal Workplace.* Ebon Research Systems, Washington, DC: 1984. 202 pp. (NTIS PB86-222213/XAB)

Other Readings

Health Consequences of Smoking: Chronic Obstructive Lung Disease: A Report of the Surgeon General. U.S. Department of Health and Human Services, Public Health Service. Washington, DC: Superintendent of Documents, U.S. Government Printing Office, 1984. 569 pp. DHHS(PHS)84-50205.

Mortality From Diseases Associated With Smoking: United States, 1960–77. Health and Human Services Dept., Public Health Service. Washington, DC: Superintendent of Documents, U.S. Government Printing Office, 1982. 82 pp. HHS(PHS)82-1854.

O'Neill, I.K., K.D. Brunnemann, B. Dodet, and D. Hoffmann, *Environmental Carcinogens: Methods of Analysis and Exposure Measurement—Passive Smoking* (IARC Manual Series, Vol. 9). 372 pp. International Agency for Research on Cancer (IARC), 150 Cours Albert Thomas, F-69372 Lyon Cedex 08, France.

Unless You Decide to Quit, Your Problem Isn't Going to be Smoking, Your Problem's Going to be Staying Alive. HEW, Center for Disease Control, National Clearinghouse for Bureau of Health Education. Washington, DC: Superintendent of Documents, U.S. Government Printing Office, 1972. 11 pp. DHEW(CDC)78-8705.

Weis, William L. and Bruce W. Miller,; Barret, Stephen, Ed. *The Smoke-Free Workplace*. ISBN 0-87975-309-9, 196 pp., 1985. Prometheus Books, Buffalo, NY.

Zaridze, D.G. and R. Peto. *Tobacco: A Major International Health Hazard* (IARC Scientific Publication No. 74). ISBN 92-832-1174-x, 1986. Oxford University Press, Walton St., Oxford OX2 6PD, UK.

Note: Documents cited as available from NTIS may be obtained prepaid from National Technical Information Service, 5280 Port Royal Road, Springfield, VA 22161; telephone (703) 487-4650.

Index